PATIENTS, POLICIES AND POLITICS

STATE OF HEALTH SERIES

Edited by Chris Ham, Director of Health Services Management Centre, University of Birmingham

Current and forthcoming titles

Financing Health Care in the 1990s
John Appleby

Public Law and Health Service Accountability
Diane Longley

Hospitals in Transition
Tim Packwood, Justin Keen and Martin Buxton

Planned Markets and Public Competition
Richard B. Saltman and Casten von Otter

PATIENTS, POLICIES AND POLITICS

Before and After *Working for Patients*

John Butler

Open University Press
Buckingham · Philadelphia

Open University Press
Celtic Court
22 Ballmoor
Buckingham
MK18 1XW

and
1900 Frost Road, Suite 101
Bristol, PA 19007, USA

First Published 1992

A catalogue record of this book is available from the British Library

Library of Congress Cataloging-in-Publication Data

Butler, John R.
Patients, policies, and politics: before and after 'Working for patients'/John Butler.
p. cm. – (State of health)
Includes bibliographical references and index.
ISBN 0–335–15647–9 (pb.) ISBN 0–335–15648–7 (hb.)
1. National Health Service (Great Britain)
I. Working for patients. II. Title. III. Series
[DNLM: 1. Delivery of Health Care – Great Britain.
2. Health Policy – Great Britain. 3. State Medicine – organization & administration – Great Britain.
W 275 FA1 B97p]
RA412.5.G7B87 1992
362.1'0941 – dc20
DNLM/DLC
for Library of Congress
92–18762
CIP

Typeset by Type Study, Scarborough
Printed in Great Britain by St Edmundsbury Press
Bury St Edmunds, Suffolk

CONTENTS

SERIES EDITOR'S INTRODUCTION

Health services in many developed countries have come under critical scrutiny in recent years. In part this is because of increasing expenditure, much of it funded from public sources, and the pressure this has put on governments seeking to control public spending. Also important has been the perception that resources allocated to health services are not always deployed in an optimal fashion. Thus at a time when the scope for increasing expenditure is extremely limited, there is a need to search for ways of using existing budgets more efficiently. A further concern has been the desire to ensure access to health care of various groups on an equitable basis. In some countries this has been linked to a wish to enhance patient choice and to make service providers more responsive to patients as 'consumers'.

Underlying these specific concerns are a number of more fundamental developments which have a significant bearing on the performance of health services. Three are worth highlighting. First, there are demographic changes, including the ageing population and the decline in the proportion of the population of working age. These changes will both increase the demand for health care and at the same time limit the ability of health services to respond to this demand.

Second, advances in medical science will also give rise to new demands within the health services. These advances cover a range of possibilities, including innovations in surgery, drug therapy, screening and diagnosis. The pace of innovation is likely to quicken as the end of the century approaches, with significant implications for the funding and provision of services.

Third, public expectations of health services are rising as those who use services demand higher standards of care. In part, this is stimulated by developments within the health service, including the availability of new technology. More fundamentally, it stems from the emergence of a more educated and informed population, in which people are accustomed to being treated as consumers rather than patients.

Against this background, policymakers in a number of countries are reviewing the future of health services. Those countries which have traditionally relied on a market in health care are making greater use of regulation and planning. Equally, those countries which have traditionally relied on regulation and planning are moving towards a more competitive approach. In no country is there complete satisfaction with existing methods of financing and delivery, and everywhere there is a search for new policy instruments.

The aim of this series is to contribute to debate about the future of health services through an analysis of major issues in health policy. These issues have been chosen because they are both of current interest and of enduring importance. The series is intended to be accessible to students and informed lay readers as well as to specialists working in this field. The aim is to go beyond a textbook approach to health policy analysis and to encourage authors to move debate about their issue forward. In this sense, each book presents a summary of current research and thinking, and an exploration of future policy directions.

Dr Chris Ham
Director of Health Services Management Centre,
University of Birmingham

PREFACE

This book tells the story so far of *Working for Patients*, the White Paper issued by the government in January 1989 outlining its plans for the future of the National Health Service in the United Kingdom. The story includes the political and historical background to the White Paper, its contents and proposals, and the actions and reactions to which it gave rise.

In telling the story, I have had in mind a wide variety of readers from various professional and disciplinary backgrounds who are seeking a synoptic and balanced view of this remarkable episode in the history of the NHS. I have therefore tried to avoid the unnecessary use of jargon, and to write in a style that will encourage the reader to follow the tale to the end. Inevitably, however, I have had to be absurdly selective in my use of source material. I consulted about a thousand references and news items in preparing the book, and each chapter could easily have become a book in itself. In consequence, the story necessarily bears a personal interpretation that is bound to be less than complete and that others may rightly contest. Yet I do believe the story is essentially true, offering a reasonably accurate and balanced account of the events that it reports. It has not been my intention in writing this book to present a deliberately partial or biased account of what has become an issue of deep political contention.

I write as one who is outside the NHS, but who has had privileged insights over many years into some of its inner workings. The emphases and interpretations in this book reflect not only the source material that I have consulted but also the extensive discussions that I have had with many NHS employees, and I am very much indebted to them for their kindness and patience towards me. I am also immensely grateful for the extraordinary stimulus and encouragement of my colleagues in the University of Kent who have helped me in all sorts of ways. I am particularly indebted to Jill Relton, without whose heroic work in manipulating the text this book might never have seen the light of day.

The repercussions of *Working for Patients* are still reverberating through the NHS and will continue to do so for many years. There is no natural ending to the story and therefore no ideal time at which to write about it. Nevertheless, the 26 months that elapsed between the White Paper's publication and the implementation of the legislation to which it gave rise seem to form a natural episode about which to write. I hope that my account is a little more than contemporary journalism, but it is manifestly much less than an adequate account of this extraordinary period. It will be for historians of the future, with access to much more documentation than I have been able to consult, to tell the full story of *Working for Patients*.

1

ORIGINS

When Margaret Thatcher disclosed, in the course of an interview on BBC television in January 1988, that an internal government review of the National Health Service (NHS) was already under way, she was seizing upon the opportunity presented by a crisis of public and professional confidence in the NHS to initiate a radical change in the service that had not originally been intended for her third term of office, and that may not have been intended at all. The Conservative manifesto for the 1987 general election had promised nothing more specific for the NHS than stronger management and greater efficiency, and the legislative agenda was already full of complex issues and replete with political risk. Moreover, the founding principles of the NHS – that it is funded largely out of general taxation, that it is mainly free at the point of use, and that it should meet the full range of people's health-care needs – were widely regarded as politically untouchable. Aneurin Bevan had warned some 40 years earlier that the NHS would be the downfall of any party that tried to destroy it,[1] and Mrs Thatcher had prudently assured the nation in 1982 that the service was safe in Conservative hands.[2]

Yet there were many within the Conservative Party, and doubtless some without, who saw in the very principles of the NHS many of the manifestations of Britain's supposed post-war malaise: the heavy influence of central and local bureaucracies, the restrictive practices of powerful professions, the absence of real consumer choice; an indifference to the quality of what is provided; the lack of incentives for innovation and efficiency; and the deadening reliance upon government funds. Those who held such views were not without influence. Within the Parliamentary Conservative Party, members of the No Turning Back Group, a small but significant repository of right-wing views, were gaining places on the government front bench and later in the Cabinet. Outside Parliament, organizations such as the Institute of Economic Affairs[3] and the Centre for Policy Studies[4] had long been preaching the virtues of private over public funding, of competition over professional monopoly, and of market forces over bureaucratic control. By 1987 the tide was flowing strongly in favour of such ideals. In June Mrs Thatcher had won her third consecutive general election and secured a huge majority in the House of Commons. Much had been done in her previous terms of office to shift the traditional boundaries between public and private sectors of service, and her new Secretary of State for Social Services, John Moore, showed every intention of extending the programme of reform to the very heart of the welfare state. In October 1987, in his address to the Conservative Party Conference, he prepared the party for far-reaching changes in the philosophy and conduct of the NHS.[5] 'We have to sweep away myth,' he said, 'dispense with sacred cows, and conduct our discussions rationally . . . Outdated ideology must not be allowed to stand in the way . . . And we will not let it'. There is every reason to suppose that the Prime Minister herself shared these views but was cautious about the political repercussions of their vigorous pursuit.[6] Studies of public opinion had repeatedly shown the NHS to be popular with the electorate, and even the existence of a flourishing private health-care sector did not weaken people's commitment to a state-funded service.[7] Unlikely though it is that Mrs Thatcher had intended to embark upon a radical reform of the service at that time, the growing perception of crisis in the NHS in the winter of 1987–8 eventually left her with no alternative.

The storm of professional and public concern about the funding of the NHS that finally broke in those winter months had been gathering for some time. Throughout most of the 1980s the government had been rather more committed than its predecessors to reining back the growth in public spending, including the NHS. While there is no single or simple method of measuring year-to-year changes in spending on the NHS, much less relating them to a generally recognized benchmark of adequacy, it was widely believed that the years between 1980 and 1988 were a period of particular financial difficulty. Between the financial years 1980–1 and 1986–7, for example, the purchasing power of the district health authorities in England had grown by a little under 10 per cent,[8] and the gap between aspirations and resources had become ever more apparent. In 1986 the House of Commons Social Services

Committee calculated that, between 1980–1 and 1986–7, the hospital and community health services in England had been underfunded by £1.325 billion,[9] and in an updating exercise carried out in 1988 the Committee found that the amount of underfunding between 1981–2 and 1987–8 was £1.896 billion.[10]

The squeeze resulted to some extent from national policies that were effected throughout the entire NHS. As the House of Commons Treasury and Civil Service Select Committee pointed out in a report published in February 1988, the revenue allocations to the health authorities had frequently been based upon unrealistically low estimates of future trends in wage and price inflation, and cash limits had been set without regard to the likely levels of future pay settlements.[11] There was evidence, too, that the efficiency savings which the health authorities had had to make, and which were counted as part of their growth moneys in the following year, were consistently lower than the government chose to acknowledge.[12] Yet the policy that had been pursued since 1976 of redistributing financial resources away from South-East England towards the Midlands and the North[13] produced a geographically patterned perception of crisis: the anger of doctors and nurses and the political embarrassment of hospital closures were greatest in those districts in closest proximity to Westminster and Whitehall. It was becoming difficult for the politicians to turn a blind eye.

The media, too, were willing reporters of the human consequences of the health authorities' attempts to reconcile expanding demand with limited growth. Throughout the 1980s the press dwelt with frequent and loving detail on the closure of hospital beds, the suffering of patients with curable conditions while waiting for treatment, and the deaths of new-born babies attributed to the lack of equipment and staff in neonatal intensive care units. Such reporting was bound to influence public perceptions of the adequacy of government spending on the NHS. By the middle of 1987 the funding of the NHS had become a major theme in the general election campaign then under way, and reports from all over Britain were revealing the dire financial circumstances in which district health authorities were finding themselves.[14] Piecemeal attempts by the government to supplement the financial allocations to health authorities to pay for increases in the wages and salaries of NHS staff failed to stem the tide of political disquiet. In the first six months of the 1987–8 session of Parliament, 26 early day motions were tabled about the service cuts being imposed by health authorities and nine debates were held in the House of Commons, six of which were adjournment debates about local problems in members' constituencies.[10]

By December 1987, as a survey conducted by *The Independent* revealed, well over 3,000 hospital beds in England had been closed through the lack of money or manpower,[15] and later that month the Presidents of the Royal Colleges of Physicians, Surgeons and Obstetricians directed an almost unprecedented lament at Mr Moore.[16]

> Each day we learn of new problems in the NHS – beds are shut, operating rooms are not available, emergency wards are closed, essential services are shut down in order to make financial savings. In spite of the efforts of doctors, nurses and other hospital staff, patient care is deteriorating. Acute hospital services have almost reached breaking point. Morale is depressingly low . . . An immediate overall review of acute hospital services is mandatory. Additional and alternative funding must be found. We call on the government to do something now to save our Health Service, once the envy of the world.

The statement was partial and incomplete. It equated the NHS with acute hospital care and it failed to specify the cuts that would be acceptable elsewhere in order to provide more cash for the hospitals; yet the publicity afforded to it by the media sufficed to reinforce the apocalyptic spirit of the time. In response, the Minister of State for Health, Tony Newton, announced the allocation of an extra £90 million to the NHS to 'meet the immediate problem'.[17] By the turn of the year the government appeared to have weathered the worst of the storm. Then in January 1988 some night nurses in Manchester went on strike; others followed suit; and the issue of nurses' pay erupted afresh as the government refused to commit itself in advance to funding whatever increases might be recommended by the Review Body later that year. The *British Medical Journal*, in a gloomy editorial, declared that the NHS was moving towards terminal decline, and called for the appointment of a commission of inquiry into the financing of health care.[18] Still the government held firm: in a Commons debate on the NHS on 19 January, Mr Moore strongly defended the government's record on health care and outlined his plans for the future.[19] No hint was given of any review of the service. But the pressure could finally be contained no longer, and six days later, in the course of an interview on BBC television on 25 January, the Prime Minister revealed that just such a review was already under way.

It was not the first occasion on which a review of the NHS had been instituted in response to perceptions of crisis: Iain McLeod had commissioned the Guillebaud Committee in 1953 to investigate what was thought to be an alarming rise in the cost of the NHS,[20] and Harold (later Lord) Wilson had set in motion the Royal Commission on the National Health Service in 1975, partly in response to fears about unjustified erosions in the service.[21] But in contrast to these two bodies, which had been chaired and peopled by government outsiders, the review announced by Mrs Thatcher was tightly controlled within the bosom of the government. Led by the Prime Minister herself to ensure that the review would not waste time on the production of politically bothersome recommendations, the other original members of the group were Nigel Lawson (Chancellor of the Exchequer), John Major (Chief Secretary to the Treasury), Mr Moore (Secretary of State for Social Services), Mr Newton (Minister of State for Health), and Sir Roy Griffiths (Deputy Chairman of the NHS Management Board).[22] The review had no public terms of reference and no formal consultations were held. Individuals were consulted in private meetings, and unsolicited submissions were received; but unlike royal commissions, no lists were published of those who were consulted, much less the substance of any advice they may have offered. The review group functioned, in effect, as a Cabinet committee and its initial objective was primarily political: to change the NHS in ways that would still the chorus of discontent about its funding while maintaining, and preferably advancing, the broad thrust of government policy for the public services.

Various options for change, singly or in combination, were available to the review group in principle. Simplest in terms of its minimal implications for structural change would have been an increase in the volume of public spending on the NHS, funded as at present mainly from general taxation. Such a solution had in effect been urged by the Presidents of the Royal Colleges in their December lament to Mr Moore, and it was prominent among the policies advocated by the all-party House of Commons Social Services Committee.[10] It may also have been popular with the electorate: in a public opinion poll published in May 1988, only 3 per cent of those interviewed thought that enough was being spent on the NHS, and 49 per cent thought that the extra money should come from general taxation.[23]

The policy of trying to spend its way out of trouble was one that the government was already pursuing through its supplementary allocations to health authorities both before and after the announcement of the review, and one, moreover, that it would continue to pursue through the annual funding cycle.[24] Yet it was unlikely that this would ever be the sole or even the principal public outcome of the review. Not only would it have run deeply counter to the Prime Minister's political instincts and undercut the government's ostensible policy of constraining the growth in public sector spending, it would have failed to address the deeper structural problems that Mrs Thatcher was by now committed to tackling. Far from dispensing with the sacred cows, as Mr Moore had promised the Conservative Party in the previous October, to seek peace through money would merely have increased the pasture land on which they could graze.

There were other difficulties, too, with this option. Simply to increase the level of expenditure on the service would not of itself ensure that the more visible and politically embarrassing problems of the NHS would necessarily be resolved. As the waiting list initiative was to show, earmarked money is not invariably spent in the ways intended, and may merely increase the cost of services rather than their volume or quality.[25] And if it was conceded that existing levels of expenditure were too low, what would constitute sufficiency? The Royal Commission on the National Health Service had pointed out ten years earlier that, however much is spent on health care, it will always provide fewer services than people want.[26] More money might have stilled the worst of the chorus of discontent, but of itself it would merely have provided a short-term palliative until the next crisis arose.

A second option open to the review group was the supplementation or even the replacement of a tax-funded service with money from other sources. The alternatives are essentially few and simple in principle, though varied and complex in their applications. Five main options were available. First, additional money might be raised through earmarked taxation on expenditure rather than income. The spread of such taxation may be very wide, for example through an increase in value added tax (VAT), or it may be confined to expenditure on products that are believed to be harmful to health, most obviously tobacco and alcohol. Although a dedicated health tax of this kind had been championed by, among others, the British Medical Association,[27] it is unlikely to have been taken seriously by the review group. A substantial increase in VAT would incur unwanted political repercussions (though the government later did exactly that, in 1991, to offset the rebates on the community charge), while a dedicated health tax might be unpredictable in its yield and would curtail the government's control over the virement of public money.

Second, additional money might be raised through changing the funding base of the NHS to some form of social insurance in which income-related contributions paid by employees (and possibly also employers) would be used to fund a national health-care system on an annual pay-as-you-go basis. Health services that are funded in this way appear to be better resourced than those that are financed from general taxation,[28] partly perhaps because people are prepared to pay more in contributions that are earmarked specifically for health care than they are in general taxation which will be used for many different purposes. There was a long-standing enthusiasm within parts of the Conservative Party for a shift to a social insurance scheme, making it a probable target for consideration by the review group. In 1981 the government had examined the feasibility of just such a shift,[29] and early in 1988 Leon (later Sir Leon) Brittan had proposed a detailed version of a social insurance scheme in which people who wished to insure themselves privately would be able to opt out of the national scheme, thereby creating financial incentives for the growth of the private sector.[30]

Third, spending on private health care might be encouraged through the introduction of tax relief on personal health insurance premiums, thus easing the demands upon the state system of care. By 1988 about one in ten of the population was insured for private health care, and about 9 per cent of total expenditure on hospital care was in the private sector.[31] Tax subsidies were available for companies buying private health-care packages for their employees, but not for individual subscribers. To allow the premiums of individual subscribers to be set against taxable income might, possibly, generate greater savings for the NHS than the cost of the subsidies themselves, although there would, of course, be no guarantee that governments would continue to fund the NHS at its erstwhile level.

Fourth, the exchequer contributions to the NHS might be augmented through increased charges levied on patients at the time of using the service. In 1988 such charges accounted for only about 3 per cent of total expenditure on the NHS, and scope existed in principle for extending them to new items of service (such as the 'hotel' component of hospital care) as well as increasing them for services on which they were already levied (such as drug prescriptions, sight testing and dental treatment).[27] The principle of encouraging those who could afford to do so to pay directly for the NHS care they received was congenial to Conservative Party orthodoxy, though politically risky. In practice, as the Royal Commission on the National Health Service had pointed out, the ability to pay such charges is inversely related to people's need for health care, and the extension of charges might therefore deter those in greatest need of care from using the services they required.[26] Moreover, the cost of granting and administering exemptions to poorer patients would erode much of the net yield from the extended charges.

Fifth, health authorities might be enabled and encouraged to augment their revenue allocations through selling their services, clinical and otherwise, to patients and to the private sector, or through sponsorship deals with business and commerce. They might also enhance their capital position through deals with private sector companies in which surplus NHS land could be traded for private development in return for help in designing and constructing new hospitals. By 1988, when the review group began its work, a start had been made in the development of income-generation schemes of this kind;[32] and the Health and Medicines Bill, which would give health authorities greater freedom to generate income and more flexibility in setting charges for private patients, was on its way through Parliament. Encouragement to health authorities to exploit the powers promised to them in the Bill was likely in principle to be attractive to the review group.

Although the deliberations of the review group were never made public, political commentary informed by the lobby system of briefing suggested that, in the early months of 1988, choices of this kind about the alternative funding of the NHS were high on the agenda.[33] The options that were considered by the group appear to have been a mixed bag. On the one hand, consideration was reportedly given to the creation of a national lottery, which might raise as much as £1 billion a year;[34] on the other hand, Mr Moore, supported by right-wing pressure groups within Parliament and outside, was said to have presented at least two plans for switching to an insurance-based system, one of which incorporated Mr Brittan's proposal for permitting those with private health insurance to contract out of the national scheme.[35] Moreover, it is clear from the eventual outcome of the review that the matter of tax relief on private health insurance premiums must also have been considered at some stage. Yet reports were appearing by the summer of 1988 that little progress was being made in these directions, partly, it was suggested, because of Mrs Thatcher's continuing caution about the political consequences of tampering with the financing of the service, and partly because of the realization that, for all its drawbacks, a tax-funded service is very good at controlling the overall level of spending. The breakthrough came in July, when the Department of Health and Social Security was cloven by the Prime Minister into its two original ministerial components of health and social security and Mr Moore was replaced as Secretary of State for Health by Kenneth Clarke. Cometh the moment, cometh the man.

Mr Clarke's appearance among the dramatis personae was to have a profound effect not only upon the conduct of the review but also upon the fate of the ensuing White Paper. He was seen to be much farther to the left of the Conservative Party than Mr Moore, and his arrival in the group ensured the demise of most (though not quite all) of those ideas that would conspicuously have bolstered the private sector. Still, however, the political problem remained of how to change the service in ways that would allay the public and professional concerns about its funding, while satisfying the personal and departmental interests represented within the group and allowing the Prime Minister to claim a further advance towards the modernization of the public sector services. The key to the solution upon which the group eventually settled, and which may have owed as much to the advocacy of Mr Major as of Mr Clarke, was the deflection of attention away from the volume and sources of money going into the NHS towards the ways in which it is used.[36] If the root concern of the public was an insufficiency of services rather than of money, it could be addressed just as well by expanding the output of services as by increasing the input of resources. The real problem from this perspective was not primarily a shortage of public money, but the inefficient and unresponsive way in which it was used. By the latter part of 1988, therefore, the principal issue for the review group was no longer that of funding but of the efficient use of the resources available to the NHS, especially the resources allocated for the hospital care of acutely ill patients.

Though much used in discourse on the NHS, the notion of efficiency is difficult to determine and elusive to measure; there is no single or standard definition. Most frequently, however, it has been used to describe the relationship between the resources that are available in any context and the services that are created from them. The greater the amount of services of a defined standard that can be produced from a given stock of resources (for example, by optimizing the ways in which they are combined or the intensity with which they are used), the more efficiently the system is said to be working. In 1983, for example, the Department of Health justified its claims about the improved efficiency of NHS hospital staff between 1976 and 1981 on the grounds that, while the number of staff increased throughout this period by 1.4 per cent per year, the number of hospital inpatient and day cases rose by 2.5 per cent per year, the number of outpatient attendances by 1.5 per cent, and the number of day attendances by 3.0 per cent.[37] To measure output in this simple way was to ignore the quality and effectiveness of the treatments received by the larger number of patients and was at least consistent with the hypothesis that, by increasing the rate at which patients were processed through the hospitals, more of them were discharged at a clinically premature stage, requiring further subsequent readmissions. Moreover, if the earlier discharges of the patients obliged them to make greater use of the community health services than would otherwise have been the case, the result might actually have been a diminution in the efficiency of the service as a whole. However, the review group could only work within the limits of available evidence about the links between the processes and the consequences of care, and if public concern centred more upon problems of access to care than upon the level of resource availability, then the goal could be realized in part by increasing still further the capacity of the system to treat more patients.

In turning its attention to the matter of efficiency, the review group may well have been struck by the paradox that it was obliged, on the one hand, to defend the government's claimed record of improved efficiency in the NHS throughout the 1980s while, on the other, implicitly criticizing the service for its less than optimal levels of performance. The paradox could be accommodated, as the National Audit Office (NAO) had earlier pointed out, by arguing that, although the service as a whole was becoming more efficient, some health authorities had done less well than others in attaining the efficiency savings that had been set for them since 1981.[38] For example, while most regional health authorities were achieving cost improvements of between 1 and 2 per cent of their revenue allocation by 1985–6, large variations still existed between regions and, obviously more markedly, between districts. The failure of many district health authorities to tackle their cost improvement programmes properly, the NAO argued, was hindering the attainment of even greater value for money in the provision of services to patients.

Examples of the supposed continuation of inefficient practices were easy to find. Many were minor (though not unimportant) matters of prudent housekeeping,[39] but others were larger in scale and systemic in nature. Substantial waiting lists for hospital care in some parts of Britain coexisted with underutilized surgical facilities in others. Beds, staff, theatre time and revenue resources did not always harmonize within districts to ensure their optimum use. Operating theatres were poorly managed, according to a report by the NAO, such that only some 50–60 per cent of planned sessions actually occurred.[40] General practitioners were referring patients to hospital consultants at widely varying rates which could not be explained by the epidemiological characteristics of the local populations, and sizeable variations were occurring between health districts in the rates at which identical conditions were being treated.[41] The turnover of staff in many hospitals was high, reflective of low wages and poor working conditions. Purchasing arrangements were fragmented. Accountability throughout the service was poorly defined. These and many other well-publicized examples of supposed inefficiencies doubtless served to strengthen the review group's resolve to act decisively; for as the Public Finance Foundation's 1988 report on the financing of the NHS concluded, 'there can be little doubt that further increases in efficiency are possible, and will need to be realised to make the best use of expenditure'.[42]

It was one thing, however, to aspire towards the diffuse goal of greater efficiency; it was quite another matter to identify the changes required in the NHS to create the climate in which the quest for enhanced efficiency might prosper. A large part of the history of the NHS has been the history of a continuing search for the more productive use of resources, and most of the major changes that have occurred in the structure and management of the service have been justified on these grounds. Indeed, Conservative governments since 1979 had already made many such changes, most notably the abolition of the area health authorities in 1982, the implementation of the principles of general management following the Griffiths Report in 1983, the introduction of performance indicators and performance reviews, the greater accountability of clinicians for the financial implications of their work, and the investment in better information systems. Each change had probably enhanced the efficient working of the service by a few percentage points, although any such effect was quite beyond the realms of empirical demonstration. What more could the review group do that had not already been tried? And how could it give embodiment to Mrs Thatcher's apparent view that, since change was now on the agenda, it might as well be radical in form?

The answer that finally emerged reflected a particular (and subsequently disputed) view of the springs of many of the supposed inefficiencies that stubbornly remained. Managers and clinicians were insufficiently motivated to make the best use of the resources under their control because neither the rewards of success nor the penalties of failure were woven into the fabric of the service. The beneficial stimulus of competition among the providers of care was largely absent from the bureaucratically controlled machinery of the NHS. If ways could be found of introducing real competition into the service without incurring the political hazard of challenging its basic principles, then several objectives might simultaneously be achieved: the output and quality of services might rise without a commensurate increase in the input of money; clinicians might be forced to pay greater heed to the costs of their activities; business principles would become more prominent and an important step would be taken towards the privatization of the NHS should that become politically expedient; substantial inroads would be made into the heartlands of bureaucratic control in the welfare state; and political disquiet with the state of the NHS could more easily be deflected away from government towards the performance of local managers. An enticing prospect indeed!

During the course of its deliberations in 1988, the review group received a number of blueprints for a competitive health service. Some, such as those from the Institute of Economic Affairs[43] and the Conservative Political Centre,[30] involved a switch from a tax-funded NHS towards either a social or a private insurance system of funding, and, once the decision had been taken to preserve the existing funding base of the service, were thereby ruled out of court. But others, involving a divorce between the acquisition and the provision of care, and the creation of a competitive environment among the providers, could still be contained within the traditional tax base of the service; and it was these that increasingly engaged the review group's attention as the year went by.[44] These blueprints, commonly described as internal or provider markets, came in various forms but divided basically into those that gave patients some choice and those that gave them little choice in the care they received.[45] In the former versions, people have an element of choice about the organization or agency that acquires the care on their behalf; in the latter versions, little or no such choice is allowed, the availability of services being determined exclusively by, say, the health authority within whose boundaries the patients happen to live. The review group finally settled upon a hybrid version, and thus the NHS internal market was conceived. The political transformation was finally complete: what had begun as a defensive reaction to public and professional concern about the underfunding of the NHS became eventually the springboard for radical change that had no direct concern with money at all.

2

CONTEXT

The notion of an internal market in the National Health Service was well developed in theory, and to some extent in practice, long before the review group began to explore its potential for resolving the funding crisis of 1987–8. It represented the particular application of a much broader set of social, political and economic ideas that developed throughout the 1980s and that gave to Mrs Thatcher's governments a philosophical coherence that was distinctive in post-war British politics. The ideas were generated and applied throughout much of western – and even eastern – Europe as well as in the United Kingdom; but the singular nature of Mrs Thatcher's vision, allied to the formidable political power base that she had assembled, ensured their distinctively widespread application throughout many areas of public and private activity in the UK.

The spirit of the times can never be captured in a few impressionistic phrases, yet a number of general articles of faith can be discerned that gave shape and direction to government policy throughout the decade. Achievement did not always match aspiration, to be sure, and greater progress was made in the application of some ideas than of others. Nor were these ideas the pure expressions of a faith that could never be compromised by earthy pragmatism or political opportunism. Yet they gave the decade a reforming energy that was to permeate many aspects of the corporate and personal life of the nation, including eventually the National Health Service itself.

At the heart of the government's philosophy lay a number of core convictions. One was a belief in the paramount importance of a sound economy and a strong currency, the pursuit of which took precedence over other aims and objectives. Social policy had always to be subservient to economic policy, for the ultimate test of government competence was seen to lie in its management of the economy, not of the social programme. Thus Patrick (later Lord) Jenkin, the Secretary of State for Social Services, was able to warn, early in the decade, that 'the government's top priority must be to get the economy right, and for that reason it cannot be assumed that more money will always be available to be spent on health care'.[1] Almost ten years later the Chancellor of the Exchequer, Norman Lamont, voiced a similar sentiment in his judgement that the rising level of unemployment was a price 'well worth paying' in order to control inflation.[2]

Another core conviction was that nothing should be done in the public sector that could just as well be done in private hands. The outworking of this conviction took various forms. Public sector assets and industries were sold off to private investors on a scale that would scarcely have seemed possible in 1980. Individuals were exhorted and encouraged to look to private rather than public services to meet their personal needs. Organizations that remained within the public sector were given new powers of trade between themselves and the private sector. And underpinning all of this was the belief that rising levels of spending in the public sector, requiring either an increase in taxation or an expansion of national borrowing, were detrimental to economic growth and individual initiative and should be held in tight rein. In the case of health care, in particular, this led to an abiding tension for much of the decade between the government's instinctive desire to control the flow of public money into the NHS and its electoral need to proclaim the service safe in Conservative hands.[3]

Supporting these core convictions were a number of other articles of faith that provided a leitmotif for domestic policy throughout the decade. One was the belief that individuals are the best judges of their own welfare and should be allowed the maximum possible effective choice in securing it. Individualism in a consumer society was the order of the day, not the pursuit of social equality through collective action. Another was a belief in the ubiquity of organizational inefficiencies and the imperative need to root them out in all their manifestations. The Civil Service, local government, education, public and private industries, and not least the NHS were held to be suffering from overmanning, restrictive practices, low levels of productivity and sheer bad housekeeping, all squandering the resources of the nation and sapping its competitive potential. And a third was the belief that this sorry state of affairs owed much to the dominant influence of corporate groups concerned more with preserving their privileges and powers than with modernizing their activities and enhancing their efficiency. The trade unions were an early and obvious target for reform, but the corrective zeal did not stop there: as the decade progressed, professions and institutions that had become well versed in protecting their traditional interests were forced to revise their attitudes and change their practices. The law, the universities, the medical profession, the armed forces, the schools, the financial markets – almost every major institution save that of Parliament itself was successively touched by the crusade to break the stranglehold of conspiracy and liberate the spirit of entrepreneurialism.

A good deal of reliance was placed in all of this upon the power of market forces to bring about the desired changes. Markets, it was believed, are better than bureaucracies at stimulating and managing the efficient production of goods and services and at delivering them to the customers who want them. On the supply side, so the argument ran, providers have real incentives to maximize the quality and minimize the price of what they produce, for otherwise they will lose out to their competitors. On the demand side, markets give expression to the ideals of individualism and consumerism by supplying the things that people want rather than those which others believe they ought to have. Effective choice for consumers and real incentives to efficiency for providers, so it was believed, are better ensured by markets than by bureaucracies, where the distribution of goods and services is greatly influenced by administrative ordinance and professional predilection.

In practice, markets must always be managed to a greater or lesser extent to avoid the calamitous consequences to which they might otherwise be prone. Consumers need protection from exploitation by groups of conspiratorial providers (oligopolies) who acquire the power to dictate the terms of the relationship. Suppliers must be protected from organized purchasers who acquire a similarly dominant role (oligopsonies). Subsidies and other forms of interference with the free play of market forces must be introduced to prevent the occurrence of intolerable inequalities. Adverse external effects must be minimized. Those who fall innocent victims to the market must be reasonably compensated. And so on. The problem is essentially one of judgement and balance: on the one hand, markets must not be allowed the freedom to produce outcomes that are economically or socially unacceptable; on the other hand, they must not be so tightly managed that they fail to provide effective incentives to efficient behaviour. As will be seen, the problem of achieving a politically judicious balance in the internal market in the NHS was a dominant feature of its neonatal life.

The outworking of these articles of faith within the National Health Service produced changes throughout the 1980s that were far-reaching and sometimes unexpected. Central government control, which might have been expected to diminish under the freer conditions that it was creating, actually intensified in certain respects. While greater freedom was given to local managers for the day-to-day operation of services, political control over the development and direction of the service increased to minimize the risk of opposition to change. Hierarchical management systems were constructed, facilitating the flow of policy directives from the centre to the edges. Performance reviews were introduced at all levels of the service to ensure that things were done in an approved manner. The membership of health authorities came under close ministerial scrutiny to reduce the chance of unwanted policies being made locally. Initiatives that were politically sensitive, such as the contracting out of ancillary services to private companies and the introduction of efficiency savings and income generation schemes, were imposed upon health authorities whether or not they were wanted. Increasingly as the decade progressed, health authorities came to act more as the agents of central government than as the representatives of their local communities.[3] As greater operational responsibility was devolved to local managers, so government assumed a tighter control over the strategies, structures and resources within which they could work.

The growth in managerialism, reminiscent of the early 1970s, was therefore a distinctive and necessary feature of the NHS as the 1980s progressed, albeit one that marked a fundamental shift away from the dominant ideologies of its early years.[4] In contrast to the enthusiasm for management which had dominated the early 1970s, culminating in the management 'Grey Book' of 1972[5] and the National Health Service Reorganization Act of 1973, the Conservatives came into office in 1979 committed to shifting the balance of power somewhat away from the managers towards the clinicians. Speaking to the British Medical Association in June 1979, the new Secretary of State for Social Services, Mr Jenkin, noted the impropriety of allowing the voice of the doctor to be 'drowned among the clamour of local management';[6] and in a policy document published six months later, the government explicitly rejected the notion of general management in the NHS on the grounds that 'it would not be compatible with professional independence'.[7] That ministers enthusiastically embraced the concept of general management only four years later,[8] and went on so to change the climate of opinion in the NHS that the managers held most of the local strings of power by the end of the decade, was evidence of the critical part that managerial solutions came to be seen by the government to play in sharpening the accountability of doctors, opening up the service to the bracing breezes of competition, and enforcing the various value-for-money initiatives mandated by the government for enhancing the efficiency of the system.

The introduction of the philosophy and structures of general management in the middle years of the decade, following the publication of the Griffiths Report in October 1983, became important for various reasons.[9] It demonstrated the impracticability of separating the politics from the management of health care. It laid down the foundations of a management culture of command and obedience that increased the responsiveness of the NHS to political direction. It gave the managers new skills and powers in planning and managing clinical services, and a growing confidence in exercising them. And it created a climate of opinion and practice that finally enabled the government to implement its plans for the internal market in the face of unremitting opposition from almost all the professional groups within the NHS.

Yet the waxing powers of the managers as the decade progressed were not acquired wholly at the expense of the clinicians. It had long been government policy to intensify the accountability of doctors for the non-clinical aspects of their work, not just by subjecting them to increasingly explicit external control but also by actively involving them in the management process.[4] This was done partly by encouraging the appointment of doctors to the general management posts created in the wake of the Griffiths Report, a move designed to increase the authority and credibility of management among the medical profession, and partly by delegating financial responsibility to doctors for the costs of their work.[10] Experiments in the 1970s and early 1980s with clinical budgeting, a device by which hospital consultants negotiated their programmes of work with the hospital managers and were then responsible for managing the budgets that were allocated to them to fund the agreed levels of work, led in the mid-1980s to the somewhat wider concept of management budgeting and thence to the important innovations in resource management.

The Resource Management Initiative (RMI) was launched by the government in six pilot hospitals in 1986 with the two explicit aims of improving the information systems within the hospitals and enhancing the care of patients.[11] Though taking somewhat different forms in each of the pilot hospitals, the initiatives shared a number of common assumptions: that cost-consciousness on the part of doctors and nurses would foster economies in care; that the involvement of clinicians in the management of their hospitals would increase their commitment to the goals of the organization; that the provision of accurate information about clinical activities would bolster the quality of the care that is given; and that the introduction of management and financial information systems would enable managers better to plan and control the activities of their hospitals.[12] In short, resource management was about a change in attitudes and ways of working as much as the introduction of particular techniques and systems.[13]

Although the creation of an internal market in the NHS was not a declared part of the government's plans for the service when the RMI was launched in 1986, it became increasingly clear as the proposals for the market developed in the late 1980s that resource management (RM) would form a central plank in the raft upon which the self-governing hospitals would sail into the open seas of competition.[14] Effective competition obliges the managers of services to know about their activities and costs, to exercise tight control over the quality and efficiency of their production processes, and to foster a corporate commitment to the organization among those who work in it. Resource management promised to do just that; indeed, it was even remarked that the successful introduction of the internal market actually depended upon the prior widespread implementation of RM in the hospitals that were hoping or planning to become self-governing.[15] Hence, perhaps, the speed with which the coverage of RM was widened before the experiences in the six original pilot sites had been fully evaluated.[16] Hence, too, the political embarrassment caused by the evidence emerging from 1988 onwards about the high costs and uncertain achievements of the RMI in attaining its original aims in some, if not all, of the pilot hospitals.[17]

Against this background of the changing landscape of the NHS, two particular policy initiatives evolved throughout the 1980s that can be seen in retrospect as harbingers of the internal market, affecting as they did the role of health authorities as sellers and as buyers. On the selling side, the introduction of schemes for the generation of extra income signalled the gradual retreat by government from the existing regulations preventing health authorities from selling their services for profit.[18] The passage of the Health and Medicines Act in 1988 effectively gave the health authorities the power to buy and sell goods, services, land, ideas and indeed anything else at commercially appropriate rates; and in the following year the Department of Health issued guidelines to the authorities on how to run their local schemes of income generation.[19] The promise was held out of a future replete with commercial potential: among the things that might be considered suitable for sale were clinical services, expertise, amenity beds, laboratory services, catering services, advertising space, car parking slots and conference facilities.[20] Shopping arcades could be built in unfilled corridors and health clubs opened in unused basements. Mail-order services were created to sell everything from bandages to stretchers, and fees were charged for measuring the bodies of those who died in hospital.[21]

Commercial enterprises of this sort were never likely to raise huge sums of money, and in the early years they fell far short of the expectations that ministers held out for them. In 1988–9, £20 million was expected and only £10 million realized;[22] and in 1989–90, a target of £35 million was set but less than £20 million attained.[23] Of greater significance than their yields, however, were the signals that the income generation schemes were sending throughout the NHS about the changing climate of expectation. The long years of isolation from, and indifference towards, the world of business and profit were giving way to a new era of entrepreneurialism. Marketing perspectives were permeating through to the soul of the welfare state.[24] The very language of the Department of Health's guidelines was symbolic of the changing outlook: they spoke of the importance of 'enhancing the image of the NHS in the public mind' and of the need for 'attitudinal change among managers and staff towards the customer centred, cost conscious and responsive approach'.[19]

Many of the income generation schemes initiated by health authorities were simply a matter of raising money by selling hospital services and facilities, or of attracting sponsorships from business and industry. But other initiatives were also taken that required a more collaborative relationship between health authorities and private companies, blurring the traditionally clear boundaries between the public and private sectors. In 1987 Guy's hospital in London, the so-called flagship of the new era, transferred the management and income of its pay beds to a private company, Hospital Capital Corporation, in return for the injection of capital for refurbishment purposes and a share of the income from the pay beds.[25] Several health authorities were later reported to have agreed deals with Bioplan Holdings for the integration of NHS and private day surgery units,[26] and other arrangements were forged under which private capital was to be used for building and equipping NHS hospitals, often in return for surplus land.[27] Managers were becoming increasingly skilled and flexible in their dealings with the private sector.

The thrust towards the generation of greater income for the NHS through the sale of services and facilities did not disturb the basic responsibilities of health authorities for assessing the health-care needs of their local communities and for providing and managing the services required to meet those needs. It was left to another policy initiative of the 1980s, contracting out, to provide the disturbance that was to lie at the very heart of the internal market.

The principle of inviting competing contractors to tender for the supply of ancillary services in the NHS was one that, for obvious reasons, was greatly favoured by the incoming Conservative government in 1979: it would subject what had hitherto been largely in-house services to an efficacious dose of competition, and it would begin to open up the public sector to commercial companies. In September 1983 a DHSS circular required health authorities to set up programmes of open tendering for their cleaning, catering and laundry requirements,[28] and financial steps were taken to ensure that private contractors could compete on equal terms with existing in-house services. By the end of 1986, 274 out of a total of 1,281 contracts (21 per cent) had been awarded to private firms, and the overall savings from competitive tendering were reported to be as large as £1.8 million in one northern district.[29]

As with the income generation schemes, the importance of the contracting out of ancillary services lay less with the financial gains that were achieved, or even with the problems that were experienced in setting and monitoring the quality standards that the contractors were obliged to follow, than with the establishment of the principle upon which it was based: that the ultimate responsibility of health authorities is not to provide and manage these services themselves, but rather to ensure that they are available when and where they are required at no direct cost to the patients using them. Authorities are responsible for determining service needs and for using their resources to ensure that such needs are met efficiently and to a specified standard; but they are not necessarily responsible for the actual processes of producing and managing the services. They can fulfil their obligations just as well by commissioning services that have been produced elsewhere (whether in the private sector or by other public sector bodies) and making them available to NHS patients through local service structures.

The principle of separating the commissioning of services from their provision (which was also proceeding in a parallel way in local government) injected a measure of provider competition into the NHS while preserving its core feature of being free to patients at the time of use. The customers who were shopping around for the best deals in ancillary services were not the patients themselves but the health authorities buying on their behalf. The principle was neither new nor startling, but its mandatory establishment in the NHS through the policy of competitive tendering, taken in the context of the other changes that were occurring simultaneously, paved the way for its extension far beyond the limited confines of the domestic services. As evidence began to accumulate of the diminishing returns from the original programmes, ministers reportedly turned their attention to other services that might be exposed to competitive tender; and they found the health authorities and the managers to be their willing allies. First, non-clinical services began to be contracted out: in 1987, for example, Central Birmingham Health Authority contracted with a private company for the design and construction of an NHS psychiatric unit;[30] other authorities contracted out their portering and transport services; and the West Midlands Regional Health Authority took the next logical step in 1988 of allowing its computer and management consultancy division to buy itself out.[31] Next, quasi-clinical services began to be subject to competitive tendering: in 1987, for example, the Paddington and North Kensington Health Authority put its entire requirements for sterile supplies out to private contract, a move described by the authority's projects manager as 'combining the value for money of the supermarket with the customer care of the corner shop'.[32] And finally the process extended to clinical services when the Greater Glasgow Health Board invited tenders for its pathology service in 1989,[33] notwithstanding the doubts that had earlier been expressed by the Royal College of Pathologists about the capacity of private contractors to maintain an acceptable quality of service.[34] By the end of 1990, a directory of business opportunities in the NHS was reportedly in circulation, detailing commercial possibilities in such areas as pathology, blood transfusion services, information technology, property development and retailing.[35]

The experience of contracting out was important in laying the foundations of a market in the NHS, partly through its introduction of the cultures and mechanisms of the marketplace, and partly through the way in which it clarified the principle that health authorities could fulfil their obligations as well by buying in services that had been produced elsewhere as by producing them themselves. A further important impetus for change sprang from the experiences of several health authorities, especially those in London and other large metropolitan areas, in coping with the financial consequences of patients living in one district and being treated in another. From the inception of the NHS in 1948, general practitioners (GPs) had had the right to refer their patients to any NHS consultant, but little had been done to reimburse the receiving authorities for the costs they incurred in treating patients referred from other districts. With the exception of regional specialties, which were funded separately, health authorities were indirectly reimbursed two years in arrears through adjustments to their target revenue allocations, based upon the national average cost of the specialties into which the referred patients had been admitted. Some hospitals, particularly the London teaching hospitals, believed that they were suffering financially from this because of the complicated (and therefore costly) nature of the cases that were referred to them from other districts. They were, moreover, losing revenue through the national policy of moving money away from health districts in South-East England towards those in the Midlands and the North, and many were finding themselves with more buildings, staff and equipment than they could afford to put to intensive use. By 1987, therefore, some of the London teaching hospitals were said to be accepting certain extra-district referrals only if the referring authority was willing to pay an agreed price, more directly reflective of the real cost of the treatment given.[36] Cross-boundary charging had begun and the rudiments of an internal market established.[37] It lacked competitiveness and it diminished the freedom of GPs to refer patients to the consultant of their choice; but London managers saw it as a foretaste of things to come. ‘At the moment’, one was reported as saying, ‘we are just nibbling away at an internal market, but I believe it has got to come.’[36]

If the London experiments amounted to a nibble, a veritable banquet was being prepared in East Anglia. Anticipating the eventual introduction of some form of market throughout the NHS, the East Anglian Regional Health Authority (RHA) offered itself to the Department of Health in 1988 as an experimental region.[38] The scheme proposed by the RHA envisaged the allocation of an annual revenue budget to the region's eight districts, from which each district health authority would purchase the services it required through contracts with its own hospitals, with hospitals in other districts, or with private hospitals. The scheme was intended to be a competitive one, the most efficient hospitals attracting the greatest share of the business. The region's offer was reportedly refused by the Department, but the project still proceeded. By May 1989 all the districts in the region were negotiating contracts with their own hospitals and units for the provision of care, and in October 1990 the market began in earnest, with real money exchanging hands under the contracts negotiated between the providers and the district health authorities.[39]

The East Anglian market was unique at the time in its territorial coverage and competitive edge, but health authorities elsewhere were also becoming skilled at buying and selling services among themselves and with the private sector. In a survey of 87 health authorities conducted in 1988, 54 were found to have entered into contracts with other agencies, worth a total of £8.6 million, for buying and selling services.[40] Most of the services that were bought by the health authorities were provided by the private sector; most of those that were sold by them were purchased by other health authorities. Services were generally bought from the private sector not because they were more cost-effective but because they would not otherwise have been available in the district at all.

Similar developments occurring in other countries were further contributing towards a collective understanding of the potentialities and problems of markets of this kind. In the United States, the growth of health maintenance organizations (group medical practices offering comprehensive care to patients in return for a fixed annual payment, buying in whatever services were needed that could not be produced within the practice itself) was generating significant savings in costs for certain groups of patients with no apparently adverse effects on their health.[41] In Sweden, the county councils began experimentally to introduce competition among public and private providers in order to increase patients' choices and to link the budgets of hospitals more closely to the work they did.[42] In the Netherlands, a number of local demonstration projects set up in the 1980s to evaluate the effect of financial incentives on the efficient provision of services led the influential Dekker Report to conclude in 1987 that 'market forces provide an answer to the organizational inflexibility and cumbersome operation of the health system in the Netherlands, characterized as it is by its high costs, lack of choice and lack of incentives for change'.[43] In New Zealand Alan Gibbs, a businessman appointed by the government to review the organization and management of the health service in that country, recommended in his 1988 report the creation of a new system in which the regional health authorities would continue to be funded by the government but would use their resources to purchase care from a range of competing providers, including public, private and voluntary hospitals.[44] This proposal, which was very similar to the East Anglian model, was said to have influenced the thinking of the Prime Minister's review group on the NHS,[45] and the White Paper that finally emerged from it bore very close similarities to the Gibbs Report. Though initially rejected by the New Zealand government, the principal ideas in the Gibbs Report were eventually enacted by the new Conservative government in 1991 for implementation in 1992–3.[46]

In parallel with these assorted experiences and initiatives, both domestic and foreign, academics were attempting throughout the 1980s to develop models of how the introduction of market competition into the NHS might actually work. Interestingly in the light of the form that the government's proposals eventually took, some of the early formulations envisaged GPs, not the health authorities, as the buyers in the market. For example, at a conference organized by the Office of Health Economics in 1984, the (then) radical idea was floated of giving GPs annual budgets from which they would pay for the cost of the drugs they prescribed and of the care received by their patients whenever they were referred to a hospital.[47] Such an innovation, it was argued, would stimulate the delivery of good hospital services at reasonable cost and would encourage GPs to moderate their prescribing and referral behaviour. If, moreover, their budgets were made up of capitation payments related to the numbers of patients registered with them, there would be a further incentive for practices to attract additional patients through the provision of services responsive to patients' demands.

Notwithstanding an extraordinarily convenient characteristic of this idea (that it introduces market forces into both primary and secondary care without disturbing the founding principles of the NHS), little further public discussion of it occurred until the final stages of the gestation of the White Paper. Instead, the torch of innovative thinking was taken up by an American academic, Professor Enthoven, whose monograph on the management of the NHS, published in 1985,[48] was eventually to exert a decisive influence over the direction of the review group's thinking.[49] At the heart of Enthoven's analysis of the ailments afflicting the NHS were the twin diagnoses of institutional sclerosis, frustrating the introduction of change, and the absence of incentives to innovation. Basing his prescription for cure in the (then) new experiences of competitive tendering for domestic services, Enthoven outlined an alternative structure for the NHS in which health authorities would receive government funds through the existing allocatory mechanisms and would continue to be responsible for providing (and paying for) comprehensive care for their own residents. Any care given to patients from other districts would, however, be reimbursed under the terms of a contract negotiated between the districts. Each health authority would effectively operate as a nationalized company, buying and selling services to and from each other and the private sector. Managers would be free to purchase services at competitive prices, to control their own programmes of capital development, to introduce innovative management techniques, and generally to run their districts in their own ways. Enthoven described his proposed system as one of 'market socialism', in which the benefits of market competition coexisted with the maintenance of the principle of free care. He was also, however, careful to set out certain preconditions for the feasible operation of the scheme. General practitioners might be able to refer their patients only to those hospitals with which their health authorities had pre-existing contracts. Consultants might be contracted to district health authorities on individually negotiated terms and conditions of service. And adequate management information systems would be required to drive the market. None of these preconditions would be easy to create.

Notwithstanding Enthoven's explicit characterization of his scheme as 'market socialism', and notwithstanding also the rejection of the concept of an internal market by the NHS Management Board in 1986 as impracticable and politically unacceptable,[50] the idea engaged the interest of the Prime Minister; and by the time the review group on the NHS had begun to meet under her chairmanship early in 1988, she was reportedly in favour of a competitive market in the NHS.[51] As the year progressed and it became increasingly clear that some version of an internal market would eventually emerge, the likely structure and functioning of such a market in the NHS came under close scrutiny.[52] Opinion was broadly in favour of proceeding experimentally, subject to the introduction of safeguards.[53] In a balanced account of the pros and cons of an internal market in July 1988, the House of Commons Social Services Committee concluded that, provided the requisite information systems and working relationships could be created, the market could

> give districts an incentive to use their spare capacity for providing services . . . provide a necessary incentive for producing better management information on costs and outcomes . . . reduce the perverse incentives by which districts which currently expand their activities incur extra costs and may then have to reduce activity in order to stay within their cash limit . . . and, within limits, achieve better patient outcomes and lower costs.[54]

Conspicuous by its absence from the debate at this stage was any clear analysis of the ills of the NHS that the internal market was supposed to treat. There was much assertion about the supposed benefits of the market, but little theoretical or empirical analysis of the particular problems upon which it could beneficially be brought to bear. Nevertheless, it was clear by the winter of 1988–9 that some version of the internal market would be the centrepiece of the review group's report, and, by the time the report was fully and accurately leaked in the national press a week before its publication,[55] the hot question was not whether a market would be proposed but the particular form that it would take.

3

CONTENT

The results of the review group's deliberations appeared in the form of a White Paper, *Working for Patients*, published on 31 January 1989.[1] It covered the whole of the United Kingdom in a broadly uniform way, albeit with nuances of style and content for England, Wales, Scotland and Northern Ireland. (If the remainder of this book incorporates the terminology that is most appropriate to the NHS in England, that is simply a matter of convenience in a short work, not of ethnocentricity.) Politically the White Paper was a brilliant document, allowing the government to please its supporters by claiming to open the NHS to competitive forces while assuring the nation of its continuing commitment to the principles of a tax-funded service that is largely free at the point of use. As a plan of action, however, the White Paper was noticeably lightweight, and even the eight working papers, published a month later, raised far more questions than they answered about the way the market would actually work.[2]

The cost and scale of the launch and subsequent promotion of the White Paper signalled the government's awareness of the need to market its proposals aggressively, not least among the NHS staff whose task it would be to make them work.[3] The launch began in a London studio among invited representatives from two of the Thames regions. Hosted by a well-known TV presenter and linked by closed-circuit television to invited audiences in eight other cities, the Secretary of State, Kenneth Clarke, explained the nature and purpose of the changes and answered questions from senior managers and health authority chairmen.[4] The show was later repeated in Bristol for NHS staff in the South-West. Communication packs containing video films, slides and leaflets were issued by the Department of Health to aid the dissemination of the message, and further roadshows were held later in the year to encourage the interest of local managers in the more controversial elements of the White Paper.[5] In April the Secretary of State wrote to every GP in the country,[6] and in the following June a 27-page booklet explaining the benefits of the changes was delivered to 20 million homes in the UK at a cost of £2.75 million.[7] A regular Departmental news bulletin was produced. As a large-scale exercise in political marketing, the government's management of the White Paper was probably without precedence; though as will be seen, the launch was merely the opening salvo in a ferocious campaign of propaganda and counter-propaganda.

At the heart of the changes proposed in the White Paper lay the principle of the division of responsibility between the commissioning and the providing of care. Authorities that are responsible for commissioning health services and making them available (that is, assessing the health-care needs of a population and ensuring that such needs are met as fully as the available resources allow) need not necessarily be responsible also for the actual provision and management of the services through which the care is given. Indeed, it is better that they should not be, for their role will not then become confused, and their judgements as commissioners will not be clouded by the influence that might otherwise be exerted over them by powerful groups or coalitions among the providers whom they employ and manage.

The principle of the division of responsibility between the commissioning and providing of services was one that had largely been blurred throughout the lifetime of the NHS: health authorities had had responsibility for both, and the distinction between them had neither readily nor widely been recognized. Yet the introduction of mandatory competitive tendering for ancillary services in 1983[8] had begun to make the principle intelligible, if not wholly acceptable, and widespread experience was beginning to accumulate in local government of how it was working elsewhere in the public sector. The 1980 Local Government Act had required local authorities to put their highway and building maintenance programmes out to competitive tender, and the 1988 Local Government Act had extended the range of designated services to include refuse collection, catering, leisure management, the cleaning of streets and buildings, and the maintenance of grounds and vehicles. *Working for Patients* had an obvious familial affinity with these developments: at its simplest, it could be understood as an extension of the principle of competitive tendering from ancillary to clinical services, the competing providers including public as well as private providers.

Since the White Paper was, at heart, concerned with effecting the split between commissioning and providing, its main proposals for change can be organized around three key questions: who should be the commissioners; who should be the providers; and how they should be related.

The review group's conclusions about commissioning seem to have remained fluid until late in their deliberations. Two basic models had been widely discussed: one, proposed by Professor Enthoven[9] and reportedly favoured by at least some members of the group,[10] envisaged the district health authorities (DHAs) as the commissioners; the other, aired most prominently at a conference hosted in 1984 by the Office of Health Economics, favoured the GPs as the commissioners.[11] In the first model, the DHAs in England and Wales (and their equivalent boards in Scotland and Northern Ireland) would receive annual allocations of public money which they would use to commission (either from the hospitals that they themselves managed or from other NHS or private hospitals) the services that they wanted to make available to their resident populations. The GPs in this model would not themselves be participants in the negotiations between the commissioners and the providers, and they would not therefore have any direct financial incentive to use the hospitals in the most efficient ways. They would be largely insulated from the financial consequences of their referral patterns, save that their freedom of referral would be constrained by the contracts that had been placed by their DHAs. In the second model, no such financial protection would be afforded to the GPs: it was they who would receive the annual allocations of money for the purchase of the hospital services needed by their patients, and they would be open to the opportunity costs facing any purchaser. The more they chose to spend on one thing, the less they would have available for another. They would, however, be free to determine their own referrals within the limits of their allocations. In this model the DHAs would be on the provider side of the relationship, responsible for the provision and management of hospital services in competition with each other and with the private hospitals for the custom of the GPs.

It appears that, as the deliberations of the review group proceeded throughout 1988, opinion hardened towards the second model, and by the end of the year Mr Clarke was reportedly favouring a scheme in which the GPs would be the budget-holders, purchasing whatever health care was needed by their patients that they could not provide themselves.[12] A possible reason, suggested by the Minister of State for Health, David Mellor, in an interview given to *The Independent* in December 1988, was the overriding need to curb the behaviour of some GPs by subjecting them to a financial discipline.[13]

> There is the whole question of looking at prescribing practices or referral practices. The Chief Medical Officer estimated that some practices referred twenty times as many patients as others to hospitals. Can those extremes be justified? We don't think it's good if people are referred unnecessarily to hospital: it's worrying for them and costly for us . . . What we have to recognise is that while respecting the professional independence of doctors, there is a duty on all of us to be able to give a clearer cogent account of what we have done.

In the event, the White Paper settled for a hybrid version of the two models. It was as though the review group would ideally have liked the GPs to be the sole commissioners but felt unable immediately to bring in a system in which they were. There were, however, vague hints in the White Paper that the scheme it was proposing for GP budget-holding might well be extended in the future. The Scottish chapter, in particular, declared explicitly that, although the scheme would be restricted initially to practices of at least 11,000 patients, smaller practices could be recruited at a later date when further experience had been gained. Later the Secretary of State confirmed that he would be looking for an increase in the number of budget-holding practices with the passage of time.[14]

The White Paper's proposals for GP budget-holding were genuinely innovative. Nothing like them had previously existed in the NHS. The Paper proposed that practices with lists in excess of 11,000 patients would be eligible to apply for their own budgets, which the doctors would use to buy outpatient care, diagnostic testing, and a range of inpatient and day case treatments for their patients. In addition, each practice's budget would also cover the reimbursements that it had hitherto received directly for part of the staff costs of other members of the practice team, any improvements that were made to the practice premises, and the cost of the drugs prescribed by the GPs in the practice. It would not include the doctors' own remuneration, which would be unaffected by the budget. Budget-holding would be voluntary, and the budgets would be negotiated individually between each practice and its regional health authority. They would be monitored by the family practitioner committee (later renamed the family health services authority). Practices would be free to switch their expenditure between budgetary headings, and they could retain and reinvest any end-of-year savings. Overspending by up to 5 per cent of the budget in each year would be carried over to the next year's allocation; persistent overspending in excess of this could result in the loss of budget-holding status. The White Paper envisaged that, initially, about a thousand practices in the UK would be eligible to apply for budgets, covering about a quarter of the population.

Practices that elected not to apply for a budget, or that were ineligible, would not be unaffected by the forced division between commissioning and contracting, but they would not be direct players in the game. Instead, the commissioning of the hospital services required by patients registered with these practices would be done by the DHAs; and, as foreseen by Professor Enthoven, the GPs would normally be able to refer patients only to those hospitals with which the authorities had negotiated contracts. The DHAs in England and Wales (and their equivalent boards in Scotland and Northern Ireland) were therefore to be the second category of commissioners, along with the budget-holding general practices. Initially, and possibly for some time, the DHAs would account for much the larger share of the commissions that were placed; but their responsibility would steadily diminish as the number of budget-holding practices grew, for the element of each practice budget that covered the purchase of hospital services would be deducted from the district allocations. The total volume of resources available for the commissioning of hospital services in each district would thus remain the same, but with the passage of time more of it would be channelled through the budget-holding GPs and less through the DHAs.

So much for the White Paper's proposals for the commissioning side of the market. On the provider side, the Paper envisaged three types of hospital competing against each other for the custom of the DHAs and the budget-holding practices: independent hospitals; self-governing hospitals; and hospitals remaining under the management control of the DHAs. The inclusion of independent hospitals, though seemingly radical in enabling public money to be spent on the treatment of NHS patients in private facilities, was no more than the logical extension of a trend that had been developing throughout the 1980s. The Health and Medicines Act of 1988, formalizing the growing experiences of NHS managers in trading with the private sector, had given the health authorities wide powers to buy and sell their services; and the White Paper was merely building upon this:

> The Government believes that there is scope for much wider use of competitive tendering, beyond the non-clinical support services which have formed the bulk of tendering so far. This can extend as far as the wholesale 'buying in' of treatments for patients from private sector hospitals and clinics . . .

Much more innovative than the buying in of services from the independent sector was the White Paper's proposal for the creation of self-governing hospitals. Any large hospital, but particularly the major acute hospitals, could apply to opt out of management control by their DHAs and become NHS hospital trusts, governed by boards of directors comprising both executive and non-executive members. Trusts would be able to employ their own staff, buy and sell goods and services, and raise capital by borrowing either from the government or in the financial markets. They could compete for both NHS and private patients, and their revenue would derive exclusively from the sale of their services. They would be accountable not to the DHAs but to the Secretary of State, who might delegate his responsibilities in this respect to the RHAs. Almost as an aside, the White Paper speculated upon the long-term implications of the growth of self-governing hospitals for the DHAs themselves: as both their management responsibilities and their commissioning functions declined, their viability would need to be reviewed and the possibility considered of wedding them with neighbouring districts and with the family practitioner committees.

The concept of self-governing hospital trusts had its historical model in the pre-NHS voluntary hospitals and its contemporary model in the chronologically more advanced policy of allowing schools to opt out of control by their local education authority. There was, however, curiously little public discussion of the concept until just before the White Paper's appearance. Professor Enthoven's vision of the internal market, which had seemingly exerted a considerable influence over government thinking, contained no trace of a self-governing hospital, nor did the discussion of the internal market in the 1988 report of the House of Commons Social Services Committee on the future of the National Health Service.[15] Yet stories were appearing by December of that year of the government's attempts to interest some London teaching hospitals in the idea, albeit a modified version in which the hospitals' fixed overhead costs would be funded directly by the Department of Health and only the variable costs covered by contracts with the DHAs.[16] By January 1989, with the publication of the White Paper still three weeks away, local managers were talking openly to the press about the prospects for self-government of their local hospitals.[17] Those in districts containing large teaching hospitals such as Guy's and St Thomas's in London and St James' in Leeds, with the capacity to do more work than they were funded for, saw nothing but hope in the prospect of self-government, but others were more cautious. 'I can see no advantage in opting out', a London manager was reported as saying, 'and I would not like to break the links we have with the local community.' 'Opting out may work for a single specialty hospital with a large patient remit', said another, 'but it is total madness for the average district general hospital.'[18]

The third category of providers, along with the independent hospitals and the self-governing trusts, were those that, for reasons either of choice or size, would not be destined for self-governing status. Though not specifically identified in the White Paper as direct competitors against the other two, the logic of the market assigned them just such a role. The budget-holding general practices would be hampered in their dealings in the market if they had no rights of purchase from the directly managed hospitals, and the hospitals in turn would lose revenue if they were not permitted to compete for the GPs' custom. Although, therefore, much was made in the White Paper of the distinction between self-governing and directly managed hospitals, with the promise that the former might enjoy a privileged access to new sources of funds, it soon became apparent that the distinction was largely illusory: all NHS hospitals, however they were managed, would be in competition with each other and with the independent hospitals for the cash-limited crock of gold, and all could be winners or losers in the market.

The White Paper's proposals for relating the commissioners and the providers embodied the commercial principles upon which the edifice was built: they would behave towards each other as buyers and sellers, the relationship being a contractual one. The contracts governing the trade in services would be agreed between the parties and would stipulate the amount and quality of services to be provided and the basis for the calculation of their costs. Contracts entered into with the private sector would be legally binding; those between DHAs and their own directly managed hospitals would be enforced through the normal management process; and those with the new self-governing hospitals would be governed by arbitration procedures aimed at avoiding the need for recourse to the law.

Three types of contract were proposed: block; cost-and-volume; and cost-per-case. Block contracts would require the buyer (whether a DHA or a budget-holding general practice) to pay the hospital an annual fee in return for allowing patients access to a defined range of facilities. The contract would specify the amount of each facility to be provided but not the maximum or minimum numbers of patients who could be referred for treatment. Cost-and-volume contracts would, by contrast, relate to the actual numbers of patients treated: in return for an annual fee, the DHAs and budget-holding general practices would be entitled to refer an agreed number of patients to each facility, and it would be for the hospitals to manage their resources in ways that would enable them to fulfil their contractual obligations. Cost-per-case contracts would be negotiated for the treatment of individual patients in circumstances that were not covered by either of the other contracts. They might, for example, be used to pay for the care of small numbers of patients referred to specialist hospitals with which no other contract existed.

Working for Patients thus set out an elegant and compact vision of a health service in which the philosophies and structures of the marketplace would be blended with the traditional principles of the NHS. At the heart of the vision was a trading forum in which health authorities and selected general practices would be the recipients of cash-limited annual allocations, supplied largely from the general revenues of the exchequer, which they would use to buy a defined range of hospital services from independent, self-governing and directly managed hospitals. The hospitals would be in a competitive relationship with each other and in a contractual relationship with their customers. Patients themselves would be excluded from exercising their choice in the market: at best, some might have a limited choice of the buyer who would be shopping on their behalf. And the traditional boundaries between the public and private sectors of care would be blurred, though political control would remain over the level of competitiveness at which the market would be allowed to work.

It was this structure that came to be known, in Professor Enthoven's terminology, as the 'internal market', though the phrase was totally absent from both the White Paper and the later working papers. That it was a market was clear; that it should correctly be called an *internal* market (in the sense of being internal to the NHS) was less obvious, since an important purpose of the change was to engage the NHS in a competitive relationship with the private sector. There was accordingly a preference among some observers for the terms 'provider market', 'managed competition' or 'partial deregulation' as more appropriate descriptors of the trading arena envisaged in the White Paper.[19] The distinction, however, proved too academic to be practicable and the nomenclature of the internal market persisted.

Around these central features of the internal market a number of buttresses were erected to hold it all in place and make it work. First, there was the imperative need to create a clear and effective chain of management command, running from the Secretary of State to the districts and units, to ensure that managers at all levels of the service accepted the new commercial principles and were responsive to the political pressures that were driving the change. At the level of central government, the White Paper proposed the creation of a new NHS policy board, chaired and appointed by the Secretary of State, to determine the political strategies and objectives of the NHS; and also a new NHS management executive, likewise appointed by the Secretary of State, to take responsibility for operational matters within the policies determined by the board.

Away from the centre, the command structures of the RHAs and DHAs and of the family practitioner committees would be changed to enable them to function more effectively as local agencies of the management executive. Membership of the authorities would be reduced and reshaped along business lines to comprise five non-executive and five executive members, the former to include people experienced in business and commerce, the latter to include the general manager and the director of finance. Medical, nursing and local authority representation would disappear, the membership composition of each authority coming almost wholly within the patronage (and therefore the control) of the Secretary of State. Among the managers, performance-related pay arrangements would be extended from the top tier to the senior and middle grades. With the implementation of these changes the NHS acquired a management culture of command and obedience more usually associated with private businesses than with public services,[20] in which those who failed to toe the policy line could be penalized in their career advancements and those who criticized it could place themselves at risk of disciplinary action.[21]

Second, the logic of the internal market required a change in the method of allocating revenue resources to the RHAs and DHAs. Since 1977, the allocations had been based upon a national formula (the so-called RAWP formula)[22] that sought to arrive at target allocations for each region and district reflecting the relative needs of their populations for hospital and community health care. The formula, which took as its starting point the number of people living in each region and district, involved the application of weightings to take account of a range of relevant factors, particularly the local demographic structure, the death rate for specific conditions, and certain social indices. Adjustments were made to the target allocations to allow for the movement of hospital inpatients across regional boundaries, for agency arrangements, for the extra costs incurred by the teaching hospitals, and for the cost of London weighting allowances.

The RAWP formula had been highly successful in achieving its objectives. At the time of its introduction in 1977, the 14 English regions were, on average, 8.3 per cent adrift from their revenue targets, with a range from +17 per cent (North East Thames) to −12 per cent (North Western); by 1988, the average discrepancy had shrunk to 2.6 per cent, and the range from +9 per cent (North East Thames) to −4 per cent (East Anglia).[23] Yet although the application of the formula had effected a striking redistribution of NHS resources away from the more prosperous towards the more deprived areas of the country, it was judged to be incompatible with the requirements of the internal market: by allowing the cross-boundary flow of patients to affect the target allocations rather than the actual allocations and by adjusting the targets retrospectively on the basis of the average costs of the specialties involved, the formula failed to compensate authorities proportionately for the actual work done in their hospitals. Authorities that were net 'importers' of patients from other regions received inadequate funding for the volume of work they carried out, relative to those who were net 'exporters'. In consequence, some hospitals received more revenue resources than their caseloads justified, while others received less.

The logic of the internal market, by contrast, required each health authority to be funded for the care of its own resident population, and then to buy in the services it needed, at agreed prices, either from its 'own' or from other provider hospitals. In this way, it was argued, hospitals that were good at attracting business could generate more income than they would get from their own DHAs, while those that were bad might lose even some of their locally provided revenue. Accordingly, the White Paper confirmed the announcement made by the then Secretary of State, John Moore, in July 1988 that by 1992 the RAWP formula would disappear and regions and districts would be funded on the basis of their resident populations, adjusted only for age, morbidity and local variations in the cost of providing services. The cost to one authority of treating patients from another authority would be charged directly through the market rather than adjusted retrospectively through the targets. Indeed, the targets themselves would become redundant and would disappear. The immediate effect, as the White Paper observed, would be to the advantage of the Thames regions (which had suffered the most under the RAWP arrangements), for the higher costs of care in South-East England would be reflected in their future allocations.

Third, in order to ensure that competition between the NHS and the independent hospitals would be fair and equitable, the differential treatment of capital in the public and private sectors needed to be rectified. Hitherto, capital resources in the NHS had usually been treated as 'free goods'; that is, no charges were made to the health authorities for the land, buildings or equipment that they used. No such freedom, however, was available in the private sector: there, allowances had to be made for the depreciation in the value of capital assets over time and interest had to be paid on the loans incurred to fund development programmes. Such charges were unavoidably reflected in the price lists of the independent hospitals, and to expect them to compete openly against the NHS hospitals would therefore be unfair. The playing field would not be level. Accordingly, the White Paper proposed an artificial system of capital charging for NHS hospitals, in which their assets would be valued and upon which depreciation and interest would be charged. Such charges would then be reflected in the prices the hospitals would set, ensuring parity of competition with the private sector and providing managers with a stimulus to using their capital resources to the full. The new self-governing hospital trusts would be treated in similar fashion, perhaps with the additional requirement to pay a dividend on their operating surplus.

Fourth, the White Paper recognized the need, among both the buyers and the sellers, for much better information systems than currently existed in the NHS, most obviously about the cost of services but also about the processes through which they were produced and the benefits they brought to the patients who used them. The promise was accordingly made of substantial further investments in modern information systems to support both managers and clinicians. In the hospital sector, the White Paper anticipated the extension of the Resource Management Initiative to include 260 acute hospitals by the end of 1992, and in primary care it promised greater investment in the development of information systems for GPs to help them to calculate their budgets, to assess the prices of the hospital services they would be buying, and to monitor the costs of their drug prescriptions.

Fifth, the market needed to be protected against the charge of placing profitability before quality of care. A key feature of the defensive strategy was to be medical audit – not in itself a new concept, but to be conducted in a much more structured manner to counterbalance the inevitable commercial tendencies of the trading arena. Audit was seen as the 'value' component of value-for-money. The principles of audit, as conceived by the White Paper, were that all doctors should participate in the regular and systematic audit of their work; that the system of audit should be controlled by the medical profession, though agreed with the local managers; that individual doctors and patients should never be identified publicly in the results of audit; and that managers should have the right themselves to initiate an audit inquiry.

In the hospital and community health services, the White Paper proposed that district audit advisory committees should be established to plan and monitor comprehensive programmes of medical audit. The programmes should review the treatment of particular conditions and publicize the findings in annual reports that might contain recommendations for change or follow-up action. Audit should be as much a feature of the self-governing hospital trusts as of those remaining under district control, and while there would be no power to compel the independent hospitals to set up audit procedures, those that did not do so might be disadvantaged in their quest for custom if the DHAs and the budget-holding general practices required a method of auditing care to be built into the contracts. In general practice, the White Paper proposed the introduction of a comprehensive system of audit within three years, based upon the work of individual practices but co-ordinated and serviced by advisory groups established by and accountable to the family practitioner committees (FPCs, later renamed the family health services authorities). As with the proposed audit mechanisms for hospital care, local managers would need to be assured that medical audit in general practice was proceeding properly and tackling the relevant issues.

Sixth, better ways had to be found than currently existed of reconciling the clinical freedom of doctors (particularly consultants) with the contractual obligations that would be entered into by the hospitals in which they worked. The internal market in the NHS would pose the curious and difficult problem that the workers who controlled the technology of production would be neither employed by the company for which they worked nor accountable to the company's managers for the technical components of their job. Yet their contributions would be vital to the company's capacity to compete effectively for business and to meet the terms of its contracts.[24] Tension between doctors and managers had existed, and been accommodated, since the inception of the NHS in 1948; but the introduction of market competition drew attention to the problem in a way that demanded action. As the White Paper put the matter, the existing arrangements, whereby the consultants' contracts were held by the regional health authorities, had

> tended to cause confusion about the nature of a consultant's accountability to local management . . . The government believes that it is unacceptable for local management to have little authority or influence over those who are in practice responsible for committing most of the hospital services' resources.

The solution proposed by the White Paper was a revision to the consultants' contract such that they would have fuller job descriptions, to be managed locally at district level. The job description should include such features as the clinical, teaching and administrative elements of the post; a work programme showing what the consultant should be doing, and where, at different times of the day; the arrangements for the consultant's work to be audited; and the out-of-hours and administrative responsibilities of the job. Each consultant's job description would be agreed with the DHA, and, in the case of new consultants, the district general manager would take a direct part in the appointment procedure to ensure the doctor's willingness and ability to accept responsibility for the management components of the job. In exchange for these concessions, the White Paper proposed that the distinction awards available to consultants should be amended in certain respects to reward management as well as clinical skills, and that a hundred new consultant posts should be created over the following three years.

No such changes were proposed in the White Paper to the contracts of the GPs, partly because they would not have the same commercial role as the consultants in the production of services, but mainly because a separate review and overhaul of their contract was already under way. General practitioners did not, however, emerge from the review untouched. Not only would the larger general practices be encouraged to become budget-holders and all practices required to participate in medical audit, all would also be subjected to new financial constraints on their prescribing. The White Paper proposed that cash-limited drug budgets should be set for the RHAs and, through them, for the FPCs. The budgets would normally be expected to be adhered to, although they could be revised in exceptional circumstances. Each FPC would then set indicative drug budgets for all the general practices within its area except for the budget-holding practices (whose prescribing costs would be contained within the practice budget). Practices that exceeded their indicative drug budgets would be open to the scrutiny and advice of the FPC; those that kept within their budgets would be able to collaborate with the FPC in spending half of the savings for the general benefit of primary care in their area.

The objective of the indicative drug budgets was, in the words of the White Paper, 'to place downward pressure on expenditure on drugs'; but it was emphasized that this would not 'in any way prevent people getting the medicines they need'. These clauses could only be reconciled in the assumption that GPs were currently prescribing drugs that patients did not need, and that this segment of the spectrum of prescribing would be responsive to the pressure of the indicative budget. The proposal appeared to subject the regional and FPC drug budgets to cash limits (albeit ones that could be revised in exceptional circumstances), but the failure of the White Paper to state this explicitly led later to a great deal of acrimonious disputation between the British Medical Association and the Department of Health about the cash-limited status of the budgets.[25]

In summary, there was a logical and even an elegant coherence in the White Paper's proposals for a tighter management structure, a revised method of allocating resources to the RHAs and DHAs, the implementation of capital charging, the creation of better information systems, the formalization of medical audit, the revision of consultants' contracts, and the introduction of indicative drug budgets. All were, in varying ways, essential preconditions for the establishment and operation of the kind of internal market envisaged by the White Paper. The remaining major proposal of the Paper was, however, described variously as 'foolish',[26] 'silly'[27] and 'ineffective',[28] having no logical connection with the internal market at all. From 1990, people over the age of 59 would be eligible for income-tax relief on the premiums they paid for private medical insurance.

That such a proposition should have figured prominently in the early deliberations of the review group was obvious and understandable in the context of its examination of alternative ways of funding health care. When Mr Clarke replaced Mr Moore as Secretary of State in July 1988, however, the review group abandoned the search for funding alternatives, and with it should logically have gone the notion of income-tax relief for personal subscribers. The treasury members of the review group (Mr Lawson and Mr Major) were in any case reportedly hostile to the idea on the grounds that it would favour existing subscribers without encouraging many new ones.[29] Mrs Thatcher, *per contra*, was well disposed towards the principle of relief, and it appears to have been largely her insistence that ensured its place in the final package.[30] The consent of the treasury members may eventually have been secured in return for the commitment to place cash limits on the allocations to the budget-holding general practices and on the regional drug budgets, thereby reducing still further the areas of the NHS immune from such fiscal control.

Yet along with the logical coherence of the market structures proposed in the White Paper there went a noticeable coyness about the level of competitiveness at which the market would be allowed to operate.[27] The competitiveness of the market was not inevitably fixed by its structure: it could, in principle, be managed and controlled according to political will. At one extreme, the market could be so lightly managed as to produce real competition, with real incentives to succeed, real penalties for failure, and real freedom for the participants in the market to pursue their own interests. Budget-holding GPs could have genuine scope to purchase care from the providers of their choice, on whatever terms they thought best for their patients. Self-governing hospitals could be allowed to determine their own staffing structures, to recruit or dismiss staff as they saw fit (subject only to current employment law), and to decide upon their own pricing policies. Uncompetitive hospitals could be permitted to lose income and even go out of business. Having created the rules of this particular game, the government could leave it largely to the players to determine the outcome, intervening only when the rules were breached or the consequences manifestly unacceptable. At the other extreme, political sensitivities could lead to such a tight management of the market as to snuff out all effective competition, rendering it a market in nothing but name. Budget-holding general practices might be allowed to place contracts only with approved providers or only upon terms permitted by government. Hospitals in expensive locations might be protected from the financial consequences of their asset valuations. Self-governing hospitals might be required to follow national guidelines in determining their prices and pay scales. The government could, in short, intervene so heavily in the working of the market as to eliminate not only the risk of politically embarrassing outcomes but also the chance of real improvements in efficiency.

The White Paper itself was non-committal about the level of competitiveness at which the internal market would be allowed to work. It was concerned more with delineating the structures than with mandating the dynamics. The evidence suggests, however, that the market was intended by the review group to achieve a level of competitiveness commensurate with the attainment of genuine gains in efficiency. The review group conducted its business in an environment that was well disposed towards market forces, and in her foreword to the White Paper the Prime Minister, not noticeably reticent about the merits of market competition, commended the proposals for the benefits they would bring. Conservative Members of Parliament to the right of the party were reportedly 'enthusiastic' in their initial responses to the White Paper, and members of the No Turning Back Group were 'jubilant' about the self-governing hospital trusts.[31] Material subsequently emanating from the Department of Health confirmed the intention to allow the market the freedom it would need to improve the efficiency of the service. A document published by the Management Executive in September 1989 averred that 'competition between service providers to offer increasingly high levels of quality and efficiency . . . will be a major incentive to raising the standard of patient care'.[32] A Departmental working paper in December 1989 noted that, eventually, 'DHAs and GPs holding practice funds will, by exercising choice, create competitive pressures and by specifying service quality, improve value for money'. And the Secretary of State himself confirmed, in evidence to the House of Commons Social Services Committee, that competition in the market could lead to the closure of hospitals.[33]

Yet there was, as the review group must always have known, a necessary political balance to be struck between the single-minded pursuit of efficiency through market competition and the maintenance of other values commanding public support. To maximize efficiency might, for example, conflict with the promotion of choice

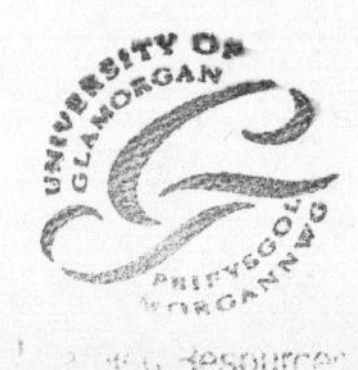

for patients and with the principle of equal access to care. The greater the choice that patients have, for example about the hospital in which they wish to be treated, the greater must be the number of hospitals offering the necessary care and the fewer will be the opportunities for efficiency gains through economies of scale and specialization. Similarly, the principle of equal access to care, such that patients in different places or registered with different doctors receive (as far as is practicable) a similar standard of care for similar conditions, may be compromised in a freely operating market in which budget-holding general practices can demand preferential terms of treatment for their patients and in which hospitals can close on a geographically patterned basis.

The government's management of its White Paper therefore came to be seen as a critical test of its commitment to market principles. Too fierce a commitment would risk the alienation of public support for the proposals; too timid a commitment would incur the enormous displeasure of major upheaval for minimal gain. In the event, the tough talking that accompanied the launch of the White Paper moderated both in tone and in meaning as the months went by. As will be seen in later chapters, not only were the controls that were built into the system increasingly used by ministers to constrain the freedoms of those who played the market, but also the rhetoric acquired a gentler and less threatening strain as the government's fortunes swayed in the propaganda war.[34] Gradually, the words and phrases that smacked of things financial and commercial were squeezed out of the canon of acceptable vocabulary as the market began its low-key life. But a market it still was, with the capacity to become increasingly competitive at the will of the government or (possibly) of the participants themselves. Having created a market, it may not then be possible to command the buyers and sellers to behave as though it did not exist. Genies have a disturbing habit, sooner or later, of popping out of the bottles in which they are imprisoned.

4

PURPOSES

The White Paper's prescriptions for action, centred around the creation of a competitive market within the National Health Service and between the NHS and the private sector, were set out in broad terms in the Paper itself and in the subsequent working papers. Prescription is not, however, an end in itself: its purpose is to change things for the better, based upon a credible diagnosis of what is wrong. What changes, then, were the White Paper's prescriptions intended to bring about, and upon what diagnoses of the ills of the NHS were they based?

The purposes of *Working for Patients* can be analysed and understood at different levels. Most obviously, it had an immediate political purpose rooted in the circumstances surrounding its conception and gestation – to quieten the rumblings of discontent about the funding of the NHS that bubbled up in the winter of 1987–8.[1] It is doubtful whether a radical review of the NHS would have been instigated at that time but for the political difficulties in which the government found itself, and only a matter of days before the review was announced Mr Moore was assuring the House of Commons that nothing was intrinsically wrong with the service.[2] From this perspective the White Paper was partially successful: it did for a while deflect attention away from awkward questions about the level at which the service was funded but only towards others that proved, in the short term, equally damaging to the government. Conservative defeats in the by-elections in the Vale of Glamorgan and Vauxhall and in the European Parliamentary elections in the summer of 1989 were blamed in part upon public responses to *Working for Patients*,[3] and a MORI poll in October of that year predicted some 1.6 million Conservative voters switching their allegiance at the next general election in protest over the plans.[4]

At a more substantive level, the objectives and intentions of *Working for Patients* can be seen as those which the White Paper proclaimed on its own behalf. While understandably avoiding any reference to its political genesis and purpose, it did contain much that could be construed as stating policy intent, ranging widely over a spectrum of precision from mere political puff to the promise of specific change. The puff comprised the grand assurances that were unexceptionable if somewhat uninformative. They could scarcely be opposed in good conscience, but neither could they be taken as promises of anything very specific. Patients would have more choice in what happened to them. The best value would be obtained for the resources available. All that was currently best in the NHS would be preserved. Patients would be regarded as people. The performance of all hospitals and GPs would be raised to that of the best. The quality of health care would improve. Hospitals would become more sensitive to the needs and preferences of their patients. And so on. A reasonable summary of the White Paper's dreamier intentions might be that they would 'enable the health authorities, within the general framework of national policy, to provide a sensitive, constantly improving service in their areas, giving proper attention to care as well as cure'. That this quotation actually came not from *Working for Patients* but from an earlier government's White Paper on the reorganization of the NHS in 1972 is evidence of the timelessness and emptiness of political rhetoric of this kind.[5]

At the opposite end of the spectrum, the White Paper proclaimed other objectives that were not only more precisely formulated but whose attainment might also be more open to verification. The package of proposed changes in general practice, for example, was predicted (either in the White Paper itself or in the working papers) to produce a glut of beneficial consequences: fuller information for patients about general practices and their services; reduced waiting times for hospital treatment; an increase in the range and quality of the services offered in primary care; greater job satisfaction for practice staff; greater ease for patients in changing practices; better information and communication technology; more systematic methods of auditing medical practice; reductions in the expenditure on drugs; increased levels of financial investment in general practice; and better management information about practice activities and costs. In addition, some potentially harmful consequences of the reforms would be avoided: GPs would have no incentive to refuse the admission of patients to their lists or to withhold the drugs they needed; they would not be subjected to coercive attempts to enrol them in the practice budget scheme; and their services would not be disrupted in the process of conversion to practice budgets. As with the White Paper's more abstract goals, few rational objections could be levelled against such worthy outcomes: indeed, if they could all be achieved through a small number of vital changes, the only surprise was that numerous other working parties and committees of enquiry since 1948 had failed to spot the way to do it.

Between the extremes of empty political rhetoric and these rather more precisely formulated objectives, *Working for Patients* set its sights upon a number of middle-range goals. There would be less variability in the way the service performed, for example in referral rates, in waiting times for hospital admissions, and in the prescribing of drugs. Those working in the NHS would experience greater satisfactions and rewards. More power and responsibility would be delegated down the management chain of command. The division of responsibility between ministers and senior managers would be clarified. Doctors and nurses would become more intimately involved in the processes of management. A closer partnership would develop between the NHS and the private sector. Local managers would have more flexibility in the conditions under which they employed their staff. And the cost of the family practitioner services would be controlled.

It could be concluded from this tally of objectives that *Working for Patients* was rather better at describing symptoms than making diagnoses. Many facets of the service were identified that were, by implication, unsatisfactory and that would benefit from the changes being proposed. Missing from the White Paper, however, was any coherent analysis of the underlying problems producing the symptoms. For example, excessive waiting times for hospital admission, which were properly identified as a symptom of malaise requiring corrective action, may have multiple causes requiring diverse treatments. Waiting times may be greater in some places than in others because of a sheer insufficiency of beds, staff or other necessary resources; because of inefficiencies in the local management of surgical workloads; because of a failure to match waiting lists in one locality with spare capacity in another; because of variations from one district to the next in the type or severity of conditions being treated; because of the inadequate management of local waiting lists; because of the diversion of consultants' time into private practice; or because of a higher priority given to non-surgical services in the light of budgetary constraints. Different causes may require different remedies; yet the White Paper was innocent of any analysis of why the excesses had arisen, why they had failed to respond adequately to previous ameliorative attempts, or why the new treatment would do the trick where others had failed.

In this sense, *Working for Patients* was an exercise in hopeful prescribing, in the manner of a doctor administering a fashionable but unproven remedy for the relief of multiple symptoms in a patient who is not allowed to know his diagnosis (possibly because the doctor himself does not know) but who is assured that, as a result of submitting to the therapy, the symptoms will improve. Historically, a good deal of medical practice has doubtless proceeded on precisely these lines, much of it probably to good effect; but as the medical profession was quick to point out, it would not do for the NHS of the 1990s.[6] Such prescribing would neither be rational nor encourage the downward pressure on costs that the government wished to see. In so far as the White Paper contained any hint of a diagnosis, it was implicit in the main ingredient of the treatment: chronic systemic inefficiency resulting from a dearth of market competition. Yet the treatment itself, though highly fashionable in certain quarters, was by no means standard, and its efficacy in tackling the multiple symptoms described in the White Paper was far from proven. Indeed, it was difficult to find any other health-care system to which precisely the same treatment had been administered, and none in which the same combination of symptoms had been observed. Within its own terms, therefore, *Working for Patients* was akin to a solution looking for a problem – or, more pointedly, an ideology in search of an application. It was not what would normally be understood as a rational process of systematic diagnosis and prudent prescribing.

Scientifically, as many argued, the correct way forward would have been through a series of carefully evaluated local trials as a prelude to national action,[7] but ministers publicly spurned such advice, claiming it would compromise the speedy commencement of the treatment.[8] In the months following the White Paper's appearance ministers did, however, elaborate upon the purposes of the reforms in press interviews, in newspaper articles, in speeches in the House of Commons, and in evidence to the Commons Social Services Committee; and these provide a further measure of insight into the government's analysis of the problems. At times such comment was refreshingly open, acknowledging that neither those who supported the reforms nor those who opposed them could really foresee their detailed effects.[9] Indeed, the Minister of State for Health, Mr Mellor, reportedly told conference audiences that the White Paper was never intended to be anything more than a framework, that its aim was to open up the debate rather than to close it down, and that if ideas such as self-governing hospitals failed to work, they would be 'confined to the dustbin of history'.[10] 'As representations come in', he said, 'we shall not hesitate to change our minds.'[11] For the most part, however, ministerial exposition of the White Paper was more committed, defending its assumptions and coherence and furnishing a third level at which the purposes of the exercise can be hazarded – that of the government's own declared objectives.

In general terms the government's argument was that the quality of care provided through the NHS was worse in some areas than it should be, resulting from inefficiencies which could and should be corrected. The reasons for this were varied. Prominent among ministerial exposition was the argument that, because of the inescapable responsibility that district health authorities had for funding and managing the hospitals within their own boundaries, resources were often used to subsidize inefficient hospitals and units at the cost of underfunding the efficient ones.[12] By freeing authorities from their responsibility for funding their 'own' hospitals and allowing them to purchase care from farther afield if they wished, fewer resources would go to hospitals with low levels of productivity and more would go to those with higher levels, enabling them to expand their services in a way that would not be possible under the existing system of allocating resources.[13] 'The use that we make of money', Mr Clarke was reported as saying, 'will be improved in the sense that it will go where the work is being done best, and where patients are most satisfied by what is being done.'[12]

Second, ministers insisted that, because the clinicians were not fully involved in decisions about the local use of resources, they had few incentives and little commitment to use them in the most productive ways. The reforms, ministers argued, would devolve more power to the local scene, would make doctors and nurses more aware of the financial implications of their work and hence more responsible in the use of the resources they controlled, and would thereby create a local service structure more in tune with the needs and wishes of the people.[14] In an interview with the *British Medical Journal*,[15] Mr Clarke said:

> The big change we're making for doctors is that we're making them more responsible, making them more accountable.

> They're no longer solely healers of the sick . . . who look to some administrator to provide them with funds. For the first time, someone is asking them to deliver a particular service, asking that they measure the quality . . . and agreeing with them that a certain amount of resources should achieve some particular results.

A not unimportant political consequence of pushing greater management responsibility on to the doctors would be the deflection of complaint away from central government. In a candid exposition of this point in his interview with the *British Medical Journal*, Mr Clarke observed that the doctor

> is becoming responsible for the performance as a whole of his unit, not just carrying out the clinical work and walking away from the rest and moaning because . . . some bloody politician is failing to provide the resources he thinks he requires. I don't think it's a very satisfactory arrangement. It leaves the politicians to sit around and take all the kicks. Government is a convenient scapegoat.[15]

Third, ministers argued that by releasing the health authorities from some of their obligations to manage institutions, they would be freer to concentrate on measuring the needs of their populations and seeking out the best ways of meeting them.[14] Although this thesis was advanced by ministers early in the debate, it seemed to acquire greater prominence, and to offer higher promise, with the passage of time. By early 1991 William Waldegrave, who succeeded Mr Clarke as Secretary of State in November 1990, was reportedly claiming as a virtue of the reforms that they would allow the authorities to concentrate not on matters of organization at all but on 'tackling such things as health inequalities',[16] and that they would, for the first time, give the authorities the explicit duty of producing a public health strategy for local populations.[17] Ministers also explained that the changed composition of the health authorities (particularly the DHAs and the family health services authorities) was a necessary precondition for them to function in this new way.[12] Hitherto, authority membership had attempted to combine local representation with strategic management, an amalgam that was regarded as unproductive of either function.[18] Many members had been unsuited or ill equipped to engage in strategic planning, often concentrating their energies on lesser matters that commanded local publicity and that enabled the scoring of political points. The new composition of the authorities, combining senior managers with a small number of lay members chosen specifically for their experience in business and commerce, would, ministers argued, resolve the ambiguity of function by emphasizing the managerial responsibilities of the health authorities and leaving the representational aspects to the community health councils. What was unclear in the argument was why the need existed for commercial and managerial acumen among the authority membership when the whole thrust of the reforms was to release the authorities from the responsibility of providing and managing services. The new role intended for them, of assessing the health-care needs of populations and marshalling the requisite services to meet them, was not obviously one to which businessmen might be uniquely equipped to contribute.

A fourth theme in ministerial apologetics, clearly reflective of the White Paper itself, was the need to correct the complacency induced in the NHS by the lack of effective competition among providers and by the impermeability of the boundaries dividing the public and private sectors.[15] 'Our aim', Mr Mellor was reported as saying, 'is to strengthen and improve the National Health Service. We will do this by introducing competition for resources.'[19] Later, Mr Waldegrave was even more explicit about the beneficial consequences of competition:[17] 'I hope that one of the benefits of the new system will be . . . the spurring of laggard departments and specialties by the fear that they might lose patients'. The stick of fear, then, was seen by ministers as one of the means by which the new competitive environment would raise things up, but so, too, was the carrot of self-interest: much was made in official pronouncements of the opportunities that would become open to the new NHS hospital trusts to improve their market position by enhancing their competitive efficiency. They would, as the NHS Director of Finance explained, own their assets, retain their operating surpluses, be able to make their own case for capital expenditure, and have the freedom to borrow money.[20] Such inducements would be crucial in motivating the trustees and managers towards better things. Moreover, as the competitive ethos gained ground, so the traditional demarcations between public and private sectors would dissolve.[21] This would occur partly because of the increased trade between the two sectors as a result of the reforms, but also because of the greater propensity of patients to shop selectively among private and public providers. Mr Clarke was reported as saying:

> I see an expanding private sector, because I think that's the sort of society we are. Disposable incomes are rising and people . . . are now beginning to want personalised choice in health care, in just the same way as they are accustomed to choosing their car and choosing their house.[12]

Fifth, ministers identified an inadequate management structure, and sometimes rank bad management, as further sources of poor care and inefficiency in the use of resources.[12,14] As a result of the reforms, ministers claimed, the NHS would be run in a more businesslike way, with the standards of management performance 'raised to the level of a well run enterprise'. In a memorable illustration, Mr Clarke pointed out that while medicine was more important than baked beans, 'most baked bean companies run better than most hospitals'.[15] 'We must improve the management of the health service', he told the House of Commons Social Services Committee, 'and we can do so reasonably quickly.'[13] Absent from ministerial diagnoses about the poor quality of management in the NHS was any clear account of why, when the White Paper's reforms were in place, the same managers who had hitherto been less effective than baked bean operatives would suddenly be able to cope with the added demands and complexities of the internal market. A hint of an answer was given in 1991 by the Minister of State for Health, Virginia Bottomley, in a speech to the Institute of Health Service Management, in which she emphasized the greater freedom that local managers would enjoy and the liberating effects that would flow from their release from the constricting stranglehold of local bureaucracies.[22] The emphasis on local freedoms, however, sat rather uncomfortably with other ministerial assertions about the need for a tightly controlled chain of management command,[12] in which the health authorities would act as the local agents of the NHS management executive. The implicit model was one in which local managers had the freedom to act only within the boundaries set by the politicians and central senior managers.

Lastly (though the list cannot be exhaustive), ministers emphasized the importance of better information systems in knowing what was happening in the service, in making more explicit choices about priorities, and, if that was how things worked out, in strengthening the claim for more resources. Mr Waldegrave actually identified the availability of more and better information as 'the major benefit' of the changes.[17] Without appearing to place quite such heavy emphasis on the importance of information, Mr Clarke clearly saw as a possible consequence of the availability of better data a more intense and better-informed lobby for increased spending on the NHS in general and on the community services in particular. 'The effect of the reforms', he told the House of Commons Social Services Committee, 'will be that a far better informed discussion will take place than goes on now. At the moment there is fog over everything.'[13] Because of the future possibility of matching money to outcome, he suggested that it may become feasible to demonstrate the value of allocating resources to the 'Cinderella' services rather than the 'ritzy, hi-tech stuff'.

Diligent though ministers were in their exposition of the purposes and intentions of *Working for Patients* and in their attempts at persuading the world to see the future through Departmental eyes, alternative and additional motivations were attributed to the government from many quarters even before the White Paper itself was published. Whether or not the attributions were sound is impossible to say, for they were largely ignored (though in some cases denied) by government spokespersons. In principle, however, it is wholly reasonable, and even to be expected, that governments have hidden agendas and covert objectives that they wish to achieve without being rumbled. That *Working for Patients* may have been intended to serve additional purposes to those proclaimed by ministers is possible, representing a fourth level at which the aims of the exercise can be hazarded.

Much of the published commentary on the government's objectives in the White Paper amounted to a matter of emphasis and interpretation rather than substance. The government's own proclaimed objectives of stimulating competition, encouraging innovation, devolving responsibility, increasing the accountability of doctors and controlling costs were widely accepted. What was disputed was the prominence they occupied in government thinking and the single-mindedness with which they would be pursued. For example, it was generally believed, in view of Mrs Thatcher's heavy personal influence over the contents of the White Paper, that the reforms were intended to produce a much more competitive and market-orientated service than ministers implied in their post-publication apologetics, a view that was encouraged by some who were known to be sympathetic to the Prime Minister's political philosophy.[23] Likewise, more emphasis was laid in some quarters upon the government's intent to attack the professions than ministers themselves acknowledged. The medical profession was understandably keen to highlight what it regarded as an unwarranted and prejudiced slight against it by refusing to consult with it;[1,24] but the doctors were not alone in seeing in the White Paper an element of a wider strategy to belittle the professions in the eyes of the people. *The Economist*, broadly favourable in its editorial responses to the White Paper, chastised the government for its 'sneers about producer monopolies and vested interests';[25] and *The Guardian*, broadly unfavourable in its editorial stance, carried an article depicting Mr Clarke as 'desperate to present the BMA as a bunch of rapacious reactionaries, out of touch with its own members and with the country at large'.[26] In this respect, the article argued, the White Paper's proposals were all of a piece with other policies designed to draw upon the public's deep mistrust of professionals, allowing ministers to present themselves as knights in shining armour liberating consumers from the deadly clutches of self-interested producers.

Beyond these matters of emphasis and interpretation, the consistent charge of a hidden agenda congealed around the theme of destabilization. The argument was not that the government was necessarily wrong in its objectives for the NHS but that, since no one could clearly foresee the detailed effects the reforms would produce, the real aim was altogether simpler: to destabilize the NHS by removing many of its lifelong buttresses and then to create from the resulting confusion a service more closely attuned to the government's will. One political commentator wrote

> The almost complete dearth of decent analysis since the White Paper was published stems from one simple fact: so much of the familiar internal landscape of the NHS will change in the government's brave new world of the internal market, self-governing hospitals and budget-holding GPs that it is almost impossible to work out what will happen.[27]

The charge of destabilization was taken up in many quarters: by the British Medical Association, which accused the White Paper of 'laying the groundwork for the future dismantlement of the NHS';[28] by opposition politicians in Parliamentary debate; and by editorial comment even in publications generally well disposed towards the proposals. 'The White Paper reforms need not result in the break up of the NHS', opined the *Financial Times*, 'but they can be regarded as a step in this direction.'[29]

Ministers and senior managers themselves lent credence to the destabilization hypothesis. Mr Mellor reportedly conceded that he had 'no idea what the NHS would look like' in five to six years' time.[9] Mr Clarke was said to have acknowledged the need to defuse the charge of dismantling the NHS by the allocation of extra financial resources.[30] And even more explicitly, the NHS Director of Personnel reportedly described the innovation of local pay flexibility in the hospital trusts as 'a weapon for breaking forty years of habit and tradition, and seeing how far back we can all push the boundaries'.[31] He was said to be quite blunt in his expectation that results would not appear until 'the present system begins to come apart'.

The government's ultimate purpose in destabilizing the NHS (if that was indeed a hidden agenda) was variously interpreted. Some saw it as a necessary and inevitable step towards the achievement of change that was widely agreed to be needed but had hitherto been impossible to effect.[32] Conservative forces within the NHS had, it was argued, effectively stifled all previous attempts at changing entrenched behaviours, and nothing short of the brutal removal of many of the familiar props would stir the leviathan from its complacent slumber. Impossible though it might be to forecast the precise effects of giving general practices their own budgets, of allowing hospitals unprecedented freedoms to manage their own affairs, and of empowering DHAs to shop around for the best deals in services, things would certainly never be the same again. Forces and powers would have been unleashed that would sweep away decades of restrictive practices, entrenched attitudes and inefficient procedures; and while none could be sure where it all might lead, the future would undoubtedly be different from the past.

For others, however, the government's ultimate goal was rather more sinister: the privatization of the NHS. From this perspective, *Working for Patients* was seen as a fiendishly clever device, allowing the government to take all the steps that would be required to prepare the service for transfer to the private sector while plausibly denying any such intent.[24] Privatization might eventually come in one fell swoop with the wholesale selling-off of the hospital trusts to private companies and the widespread introduction of tax relief on personal private health insurance premiums; but it would be more likely to result from a steady process of attrition from the public sector as the long-term effects of the changes began to bite. In the course of time and with their growing experience of behaving as if they were commercial enterprises, the hospital trusts might naturally come to want full independence.[29] The budget-holding general practices might come under pressure from the insurance companies to encourage their patients to take out personal policies as a way of reducing the calls on the practice budget.[33] The government might encourage the trend by introducing vouchers or progressively lowering the age limit of eligibility for tax relief on personal insurance premiums.[34] And the health authorities, having lost most of their functions and many of their best managers to the trusts, would be weakly placed to prevent the erosion.[29] 'Such developments may not be on the agenda today', remarked an editorial in the *Financial Times*, 'but the right-wing think-tanks which produced the ideas behind . . . the White Paper were well aware that it might end up destabilising the NHS.'[34]

A somewhat different scenario was articulated by David Owen, a former Labour Minister of State for Health.[35] While aligning himself with the view that a hidden agenda existed to destabilize the NHS to the benefit of the private sector, he saw its eventual purpose as the deliberate creation of a bipartite service in which the wealthiest 40 per cent of the population would be enabled and encouraged to seek their health care privately, leaving the remainder under the care of a cheaper state system. The change would occur as people became increasingly dissatisfied with the poor quality of care available in the NHS and as the introduction of commercial principles into the service laid it open to opportunistic invasion by the private sector. Within perhaps ten years (election results permitting), the same point would have been reached which, 50 years earlier, had prompted the thinking that led to the creation of the NHS.

The concern expressed about a hidden agenda of privatization (whether by design, stealth or accident) was not unfounded. The nation had been ceaselessly lectured by Mrs Thatcher on the virtues of the private market, and there were few grounds for supposing that anything short of electoral jeopardy would cause the tide of privatization to turn at the threshold of the NHS. The belief that the government was laying down the framework for a private health-care system, to be activated at a future moment of political acceptability, was wholly in accordance with the expectations that the Prime Minister herself had raised. Yet ministers were quick to deny any such plan, doubtless because of the unmistakable warnings emerging from the opinion polls of the electoral hazard that such a move would incur. Mr Clarke did concede that, had it been his intent to privatize the NHS, the reforms of the White Paper would have been a necessary first step in the process;[12] but otherwise he and his colleagues, including the Prime Minister, repeatedly rebutted all accusations of any such intent.[36]

The issue would not easily die, however, and for a very long time it formed one element of a vigorous propaganda battle that the government never really won. By the middle of March 1989, some six weeks after the White Paper's birth, Sir Gerard Vaughan, a former Conservative Minister of State for Health, was reportedly warning Mr Clarke of the widespread public belief that to become a self-governing hospital trust meant going over to the private sector, and urging him to 'do more to destroy the myth that we are privatising the NHS'.[37] In response, the Secretary of State wrote to all Conservative MPs denying the government's intention to privatize the service and urging them to counter 'misinformation' by opposition parties, trade unions and interest groups.[38] Prophetically, Mr Clarke warned his colleagues to 'expect a mounting attack on the proposals'. In this he was wholly correct.

5

DISSENT

The publication of *Working for Patients* sparked off a battle of propaganda and counter-propaganda that was remarkable for its scale and cost, for the furious intensity and acrimony of its conduct, and for the levels of personal vilification to which it sometimes descended. Rarely can a social policy initiative by a British government have evoked such costly and widespread dissent, ultimately to such little effect. Prominent among the hostile voices were those of the doctors, individually to the extent that their contracts permitted them to be so and collectively through their professional organizations; but they were by no means lone voices. Other professions within the NHS, the trade unions, patients' organizations, charities, churches, think-tanks, health authorities, and political groupings within Parliament and outside were all caught up at one time or another in the persistent whirlwind of critical opinion that raged around the White Paper. It would be almost impossible to overemphasize the breadth and depth of the anxiety and concern that was evoked and that seemed likely at one stage to deal a mortal blow to the government's aspirations for the NHS if not to the government itself.

For its part, the government tried to seize the early initiative through the expensive and well-coordinated campaign that attended the launch of the White Paper. Anticipating the antagonism that it would arouse, and seeking to take the wind out of the opponents' sails, the launch was accompanied by media-style presentations, by the dissemination of explanatory material, and later by letters to the doctors and leaflets to the people. Yet if the intention was indeed to scupper the flotilla of opposition before it could even set sail, the government's campaign must be counted a failure. Well before the publication date the British Medical

Association (BMA) was laying plans, costed provisionally at up to £3 million, to fight any proposals in the White Paper that might, in the Association's view, adversely affect the quality of patient care,[1] and the General Medical Services Committee (representing the interests of the general practitioners) resolved unanimously in mid-January 1989 that any threats to the standard of care in general practice would be met with 'strong professional resistance'.[2] Within 24 hours of the White Paper's publication, not only the BMA but also the Royal College of Nursing (RCN), the Chartered Society of Physiotherapists, the Royal College of Midwives, the Association of Community Health Councils, the Patients' Association, the College of Health, Age Concern, the National Union of Public Employees, the Confederation of Health Service Employees, the General and Municipal Workers' Union, the Trades Union Congress and the Labour Party had all issued preliminary statements critical of aspects of it.[3] Setting the tone for the subsequent war of words, the Secretary of State, Mr Clarke, retorted that 'the BMA, in my unbiased opinion, has never been in favour of any change of any kind on any subject whatsoever for as long as anyone can remember'.[4]

By early March the Council of the BMA had resolved to campaign, at whatever cost, against most of the key proposals including self-governing hospital trusts, general practice budget-holding, and the concept of an internal market.[5] Openly critical though some doctors were of the stance the BMA was taking,[6] most appeared to support their Association's opposition to the government's proposals, many GPs even regarding the White Paper as a resignation issue.[7] Meetings in Leeds, Birmingham, Sheffield and elsewhere attracted unprecedentedly large numbers of doctors to pass angry and critical resolutions.[8] Temperatures rose as the Minister of State for Health, Mr Mellor, signalled the government's determination to resist the obstructionist tactics of the BMA.[9] 'No man at the BMA can be a Doctor No on this matter' he said – a remark that caused him to be likened by a senior BMA official (to his subsequent deep regret) to Dr Joseph Goebbels. Mr Clarke declared himself anxious to moderate the recriminations, but succeeded in enraging the doctors still further in observing in the course of a speech at the Royal College of General Practitioners that he 'wished the more suspicious of our GPs would stop feeling nervously for their wallets every time I mention the word "reform"'.[10]

By the beginning of April the BMA had printed 11 million leaflets for distribution to patients through Britain's 32,000 family doctors, mobilizing public opinion against four of the key changes proposed in the White Paper.[11] The leaflets, described by the BMA as an attempt to counter the government's own propaganda material, posed a series of somewhat loaded questions: If your doctor runs out of money, who will prescribe for you when you are ill? Don't you deserve more time when you need it? Do you want the cheapest treatment or what is best for you? The Association's tactics were described by Mr Clarke as 'disgraceful' and 'distressing' and the leaflets as 'alarmist nonsense'; but the chairman of the BMA Council responded that 'it will be interesting to see if patients trust us more than the politicians'.

The RCN was also mobilizing public opinion against the White Paper by this time, expressing 'grave concern' about its damaging impact upon the quality and continuity of care.[12] At the College's annual congress at Blackpool early in April its Council was instructed to 'plan, implement and sustain a strategy to uphold the NHS and promote policies which address the health care needs of the nation'.[13] The White Paper, in the view of the RCN, undermined the principles and effectiveness of the NHS and placed at risk most of the progress that had been made since 1948.

Much of the early medical running had been made by the GPs, perhaps because they were in any case locked in dispute with Mr Clarke over the contents of their new contract; but the hospital doctors were not far behind. The BMA's Hospital Junior Staff Committee passed a resolution at a meeting in March that *Working for Patients* could not and would not improve patient care;[14] consultants in the six pilot hospitals in the Resource Management Initiative were said to be unenthusiastic about the reforms;[15] and the Joint Consultants' Committee of the BMA warned of 'real risks to patient care' in the White Paper.[16] The BMA prepared Britain's 18,500 consultants in April to resist the pressure from managers to nominate their hospitals as candidates for self-government,[17] and the Association's Central Committee for Hospital Medical Services announced its plans to monitor the pressures towards self-government in every hospital and to keep the consultants informed of national developments.[18] By mid-April 1989 the formal line-up of medical opposition was complete.

The government and its supporters hit back. A Commons motion was tabled regretting the BMA's action in using the GPs to 'present a biased view of the White Paper' and questioning 'the morality and ethics of an approach which is causing grave and unnecessary worry to very many elderly people when visiting their doctor'.[19] In response to questions in the House, Mr Clarke dismissed as 'scurrilous nonsense' the BMA's claim that patient care would be harmed by the proposals.[20] 'It is', he said, 'a long time since I came across a trade union that is prepared to spend millions of pounds of its members' money on spreading untruths.' If this was an attempt to discredit the BMA's leaders among the general membership, it failed. A special meeting of the Conference of Local Medical Committees in April, nominally representing the country's 32,000 GPs, unanimously condemned the proposed changes,[21] in the process shouting down one of their number who bravely suggested that the BMA's leaflet campaign may have been a tactical mistake.[22] Mrs Thatcher repeated the charge against the GPs of spreading false propaganda, but to little effect: at a special representative meeting of the BMA in May, several motions were passed that were hostile to almost all the major proposals in *Working for Patients*.[23] They would, the meeting believed, restrict the choices available to patients, reduce the standard of health care provided, damage the trust between doctor and patient, militate against the World Health Organization's targets for the reduction of health inequalities by the year 2000, disproportionately emphasize the acute services, and lead to unacceptable regional variations in the availability and quality of care. If such beliefs were indeed well founded, then precious little of value would remain from the government's proposals.

The action intensified. Doctors were advised by the BMA not to co-operate in implementing the proposals, and a £600,000 newspaper campaign was launched.[24] Built around the slogan that the NHS was underfunded, undermined and under threat, one advertisement boldly proclaimed the new spirit of competition to which it claimed Mr Clarke was now committed: 'the health of the patient versus the cost of the treatment'. Another warned patients that they could expect to be treated like cans of 'Clarke's processed peas'. Mr Clarke condemned the campaign as 'misleading and unscrupulous',[25] but it was followed in June by the release of a video film, involving stars from popular television serials, for showing in GPs' waiting rooms, and in July by a roadside poster campaign.[26] One of the posters, bearing the picture of a steamroller, was captioned: 'Mrs Thatcher's plans for the NHS'. Another, depicting a lonely woman in a hospital bed, declared that 'it's not a local anaesthetic if the hospital is 50 miles away'. And a third, carrying a photograph of Mr Clarke, posed the rhetorical question: 'What do you call a man who doesn't take medical advice?'

The poster display, which brought the BMA's expenditure on propaganda to nearly £2 million in the first six months of its campaign, attracted some critical response from doctors; but by the summer of 1989 the Association and its allies were widely regarded as winning the propaganda battle.[27] The medical and cognate professions had maintained a united front of opposition; the doctors had used their privileged contacts with their patients to spread their own particular messages; the leaders of the BMA were using their extensive experience of political strategy to telling effect; and the Association's press office was feeding the national media with information and opinion that was favourable to the doctors' case. The Department of Health, by contrast, was suffering from a crisis of morale and an excess of pressure. Its senior managers were said to be hard-pressed to maintain the different initiatives required by the White Paper; ministers were still locked in a damaging and unproductive confrontation with the GPs over their new contract; and Conservative backbench Members of Parliament were reportedly becoming nervous at the lack of apparent progress.[28] To crown the government's discomfiture, the National Audit Office warned that district health authorities would be unable to engage in the kind of sophisticated financial management required to operate the internal market;[29] and the House of Commons Social Services Committee, in its first official pronouncement on *Working for Patients*, dismissed the government's timetable as unrealistic and warned of the damage that the proposals might inflict upon the NHS.[30]

The screw of opposition continued to tighten. The BMA and later the General Medical Services Committee sent leaflets to every GP warning of the damaging effects that practice budgets would inflict on patient care.[31] A legal challenge, led by a professor from Guy's hospital, was mounted against Mr Clarke for allegedly using public funds to implement the White Paper's proposals before the enabling legislation had been passed by Parliament.[32] A federation of professional and public organizations was formed to oppose the intended legislation in the name of preserving the NHS.[33] And an embryonic political party (the NHS Supporters Party) was launched in the Prime Minister's own constituency to fight on the single issue of *Working for Patients*.[34]

By January 1990 the BMA's campaign expenditure had risen to £2.5 million; but it was at about this time that the first signs became apparent of a paradox that was eventually to cause much anguish within the Association. The realization was gradually dawning that while the propaganda battle was being won, the war itself was being lost. Of the former the evidence was reasonably clear. Medical, political and other opposition to the reforms continued unabated up to and beyond the day appointed for their implementation in 1991, and it carried public opinion with it. Even in the summer of 1991, three months after the enabling Act had come into force, a poll by NOP found that half of those questioned disagreed with the proposition that the reforms would lead to a better health service, and only a quarter agreed.[35] Yet for all its apparent success in wooing the hearts and minds of the people, neither the BMA nor its assorted fellow-travellers in protest were able to halt the relentless process of implementation. Strenuously and expensively though it had fought, the Association's senior officers were being forced to concede early in 1990 that little of substance had been achieved.[36] The National Health Service and Community Care Bill, embodying most of the important elements of *Working for Patients*, had begun its passage through Parliament and seemed likely to be implemented without substantial amendment. Hundreds of general practices were reportedly showing an interest in holding their own budgets and scores of hospitals in seeking trust status. Consultants were facing up to the dilemma that, however unacceptable they might find the proposals, they would yet have to implement them when they became law.[37] The Council of the BMA could merely fulminate against Mr Clarke's inflexible responses to its suggestions and his refusal to contemplate alternative solutions.[36]

Organized pressure continued to be exerted, though now more in hope than in expectation of amending the government's will. The BMA launched another offensive in the summer of 1990, and in the autumn it leafleted half a million households in five areas where strong local campaigns had been organized to oppose the transformation of local hospitals into trusts.[38] In response, Mr Clarke urged all hospitals actively to consider the merits of self-governing status;[39] but by then he had little to fear. The legal action against him had failed;[40] the NHS Supporters Party, though fizzling briefly, had failed to achieve electoral success; and the Bill had completed its passage through Parliament with surprisingly little opposition. Eager managers were preparing for its implementation. By October 1990 the Council of the BMA was accepting the inevitability of self-governing hospital trusts[41] and in December the first 57 trusts were unveiled. In April 1991 the first 306 budget-holding general practices were named. By the summer of 1991, with the second wave of trust hospitals and budget-holding practices in the pipeline, the struggle had effectively been lost and the recriminations had begun. In the early and optimistic days of the campaign, when the aim had been to halt the reforms in their tracks, the BMA's purposes had been clear and its morale high. By the middle of 1991 its position was more dishevelled, being likened in an editorial in the *British Medical Journal* to that of a bull that had charged the toreador, missed, and now did not know what to do.[42] For want of any clearer vision, it rounded on its leadership, criticizing the performance of its chairman.[43] While continuing to condemn the reforms, the Association's Annual Representative Meeting in July 1991 resolved to pursue its interests through constructive dialogue with the government, not through further confrontation.[44] The chairman pledged that opposition would continue, but the grounds on which it was to be fought were now less clear. A vast and extraordinarily imaginative campaign had largely failed in its primary purpose of persuading the government to seek a second opinion about its intentions for the NHS.

The anger and bitterness of the doctors, and perhaps also of the other groups of NHS employees, can be understood in part as a natural response to the perception of threat.[45] It was clear from the outset that, if implemented in anything approaching their full measure, the proposals in *Working for Patients* would substantially affect the circumstances in which many of the caring professions worked. Restrictive practices might be exposed in the searching light of competition, political influence might wane in the face of the resurgent managerialism, and the consultants' opportunities for lucrative work in the private sector might diminish.[46] Any such far-reaching threat was bound to stimulate principled opposition, especially when, as here, the full extent of the effects could not be foreseen. Yet the opposition came not only from those with self-interests to protect. A good deal of press commentary was agnostic or even hostile towards many of the proposals. Voluntary organizations, including many that represented the interests of various groups of patients, were deeply worried.[47] The mainstream Christian churches preached their alarm.[48] The National Consumer Council[49] and the Office of Health Economics[50] published their reservations. The Institute of Economic Affairs was unhappy.[51] Public opinion, as expressed through polls that were regularly conducted and published throughout 1989,[52] 1990[53] and 1991,[35] consistently and strongly disapproved of most of the key proposals, including particularly those for self-governing hospital trusts and budget-holding general practices. And the opposition parties in

Parliament maintained a persistent and highly publicized barrage of opposition to almost everything the government said and did, the Labour shadow Secretary of State, Robin Cook, being every bit as visible and audible as Mr Clarke.

In the face of the scale and intensity of the institutional and organized opposition to the government's plans, it is easy to forget (and therefore important to stress) the positive responses that the White Paper elicited. Some parts of it were accepted and even welcomed in many quarters, and many parts were accepted in some quarters. Understandably, the warmest responses came from those with the most to gain. The private health-care sector, though cautious about the short-term threat of new competition, generally welcomed the long-term prospect of gaining access to new markets.[54] Many NHS managers also foresaw a rosy future. Those who were likely in due course to become chief executives of hospital trusts were obviously enthusiastic about that particular proposal,[55] but managers without such prospects were also well disposed towards those aspects of the White Paper that held the promise of enhancing their power and easing their difficulties: the closer relationship between work and funding, the release of local management from the supposed shackles of bureaucracy, the requirement for greater management accountability by doctors, and particularly the separation of the commissioning from the providing of services, thereby freeing the health authorities from political dominance by providers.[56]

The medical profession, too, was by no means uniformly or undiscriminatingly hostile to the government's designs. Some of the White Paper's proposals, especially those relating to medical audit and information technology, were well and widely received; and even the more controversial parts found favour with some (perhaps many) doctors. A straw poll of 60 GPs, published within a few days of *Working for Patients*, found almost a third believing that patients would gain from the proposals and over half in favour of indicative drug budgets.[57] One named doctor was reported as saying that she 'could not wait to get her hands on a GP budget'. Subsequent regular polls of the opinions of GPs revealed a consistent and sizeable minority support for the government's actions. Consultants also aired their enthusiasms in public: an obstetrician expected an increase in the excellence of care and a better service all round,[58] and a paediatrician thought that the self-governing trusts would enhance the efficient management of care.[59] Medical support for the White Paper began to organize itself. In November 1989 the Health Reform Group, composed largely but not exclusively of doctors, was formed to support the principles of the White Paper.[60] It was attacked by the BMA as 'small and unrepresentative', but its views were by no means unshared, and they found support in influential places. The soon-to-be-appointed editor of *The Times* proclaimed the White Paper's innovations to be 'sensible';[61] the chairman of the National Association of Health Authorities and Trusts thought that they would yield 'a great deal of benefits for patients';[19] and several prominent academics were among those prepared to see good as well as bad in the White Paper.

Nevertheless, the overwhelming tenor of the published responses to *Working for Patients* was critical and hostile. What, then, was the fuss all about, and why did it finally fail to deflect the government from its chosen path of action?

The grounds upon which the opposition to *Working for Patients* was founded cannot easily be charted. They were varied and often inconsistent; they shifted with the passage of time and the tide of events; they differed in their nature and purpose; and they were frequently as inarticulately expressed as those that were charged to be underlying the White Paper. Ministers were to some extent justified in pointing out, in the summer of 1989, that for all the vocal dissent against *Working for Patients*, few realistic alternative suggestions had yet emerged.[62] The taxonomy of protest in this chapter and the next may give a measure of order to the story but it cannot hope to do justice to the rich diversity and complex patterning of the verbal games and linguistic manoeuvrings in which the assorted antagonists were caught.

The first point to be made is that few of the critics were arguing publicly for the preservation of the status quo. The government's assertions of the need for change in the NHS were never seriously challenged. Indeed, as the events recounted in Chapter 1 have shown, much greater concern about the parlous state of the NHS was expressed outside government than within it in the months leading up to the establishment of the review group in January 1988. Nor was there any great opposition to most of the White Paper's ostensible objectives for change. The government's expressed goals of greater efficiency in the use of resources, higher standards of clinical care, greater choice for patients, reductions in waiting times for treatment, closer alignments between resources and outputs, and the more intimate involvement of staff in the local management of services could scarcely be opposed by anyone claiming commitment to a better health service. Indeed, the BMA, at its Special Representative Meeting in May 1989, specifically endorsed what it regarded as five of the central aims of *Working for Patients*: that paramount attention should be given to meeting the needs of patients; that the NHS should continue to be funded from general taxation and available without a test of means; that patient choice should be extended; that those who provided services should have responsibility for day-to-day decisions about operational matters; and that health authorities should be responsible for ensuring the provision of a comprehensive range of good and efficient services.[23]

Not only were most of the ostensible aims of the White Paper acceptable, some of the proposed ways of achieving them also found favour among its critics. In particular, the proposals for the formalization and extension of medical audit, and for further investment in information systems and technology, were immediately applauded in many quarters, including BMA House. In March 1989 the Council of the BMA formally welcomed the government's recognition of the importance of audit,[63] and so, too, did the Royal College of Physicians,[64] the Local Medical Committees (provided it was used as an educational rather than a managerial tool),[21] and the Royal College of General Practitioners. The Conference of Royal Medical Colleges, in a sober and unemotive pamphlet published in July 1989, highlighted several of the White Paper's proposals that were likely to improve the NHS, including, in addition to the development of audit, the extension of the RMI, the introduction of competitive contracts for a very limited range of services such as elective surgery, and the principle of delegated management.[65] Even the BMA, having been self-consciously aware at its Special Representative Meeting in May 1989 of its failure to have articulated its own alternative programme of reform,[23] had rectified the deficit by September; but its seven-point plan of action bore many close linguistic resemblances to *Working for Patients*, including an extension of resource management, allowing money to follow patients to the purveyors of care, developing medical audit, increasing the efficient use of NHS resources, and emphasizing the prevention of disease and the promotion of health.[66]

So much for the precincts of consensus. The first substantive plank in the raft of opposition comprised the White Paper's sins of omission. Foremost among these was the charge that it failed entirely to address the problem of funding the NHS. If there was one single issue that united the assorted groups of protesters, including even the NHS managers, it was that the endemic underfunding of the service, and the broader issue of how it could adequately be funded, were entirely ignored. Repeatedly throughout 1989 motions were passed at conferences and congresses noting the financial crisis that had given rise to the review in the first place, regretting the government's unwillingness to fund the NHS at a level commensurate with that required for a modern health-care system, and condemning the White Paper's failure to offer any prospect of improvement. Such motions would, of course, be expected to emanate from associations of NHS employees since this would be in their interests; but the image of an underfunded NHS was held more widely than that, including among its subscribers the House of Commons Social Services Committee,[67] the National Association of Health Authorities,[68] the King's Fund Institute,[69] the Chartered Institute of Public Finance and Accountancy,[70] and many commentators and leader-writers. For its part, the government doggedly defended the view that a great deal of public money was already being spent on the NHS, that more would be forthcoming, and that one effect of the reforms might be a strengthening of the claims for increased spending.

Issues about the funding of the NHS were not, however, the only lacunae in the White Paper that stirred the fires of opposition. Widespread concern was expressed about the Paper's absolute silence on community care. The Griffiths Report on the future of the community services had been published in 1988,[71] and the government had hinted of its sensible intention to blend its responses to Griffiths into its wider plans for the NHS.[72] Yet nothing of this intention permeated into the White Paper: it was seen to be unduly obsessed with the financing of the hospitals (and acute hospitals at that), with no clear proposals for the co-ordinated development of hospital and community care. Ministers appeared to have no real defence to the charge that their proposals offered little promise of better times ahead for elderly people, for those with physical or mental handicaps, or for patients with chronic illness. Indeed, it was argued that elderly patients would actually lose out if the market diverted resources away from the many local hospitals that had developed a fast and effective assessment of the needs of older people and a locally co-ordinated programme for their post-hospital care and rehabilitation.[73]

A third sin of omission from the White Paper, causing prolonged anxiety among the medical and educational communities, was the scant attention it supposedly gave to teaching and research. A brief reference in the White Paper to the government's 'firm commitment to maintaining the quality of medical education and research' and a more elaborate statement in the second Working Paper failed to satisfy the medical academics of the government's forethought in protecting these activities from the predations of the market. Thus, the Standing Committee on Postgraduate Medical Education expressed concern that the new entrepreneurial management systems could suppress educational activity, that the freedom of the hospital trusts to set their own conditions of appointment for medical staff could jeopardize the training schemes for junior doctors, and that the quest of GPs for larger lists could deflect them from their educational responsibilities as trainers.[74] Similar fears were expounded by the Conference of Royal Medical Colleges in a constructive paper which also remarked upon the need to protect the funding of those areas of basic medical research that may not have much short-term commercial value.[65]

Anxieties about these and other perceived omissions from the White Paper were prominent among the fabric of concern; but if a storm was raised by what the Paper omitted, a hurricane was provoked by what it included. For at the heart of the symphony of protest there was suspicion and scepticism over the central claim of the White Paper – that many of the symptoms of malaise in the NHS were those of chronic systemic inefficiency resulting from a dearth of market competition, and that these were curable only through the injection of an efficacious dose of commercial principles.

6

PROPHECIES

Since nobody could really judge the long-term effects of the reforms the government was proposing (as Mr Mellor candidly conceded[1]), the edifice of critical comment that was constructed around the White Paper was as much the result of ingenuity and imagination as of grounded analysis. Some of the worst fears of the critics proved in the short term to be well founded, but others failed to materialize. Nevertheless the essence of the debate is worth recapturing, since it defined the climate of opinion and pressure within which the government pursued its aims both before and after the passage of the enabling legislation in 1990.

The symphony of protest about the competitive market prescribed in the White Paper was arranged around four main themes: that market competition would be bad in principle; that it would be unworkable in the particular form mandated by the White Paper; that, even if it were workable, the market would be structured in a way that would frustrate the achievement of many of its own objectives; and that it would damage or even destroy many of the best features of the NHS.

The first theme, that market competition would be bad in principle as the organizational basis of a modern health-care service, drew heavily upon recent American experience revealing bane as well as boon in its system.[2] Various steps had been taken in the USA throughout the 1980s to sharpen the market competitiveness of health care, partly in order to curb what was seen to be a damagingly rapid increase in the cost of care.[3] Cost-sharing arrangements had been extended to make patients more aware of the real cost of their treatment; legislation had been passed to limit anti-competitive behaviour among providers; and new forms of managed health-care provision, such as health maintenance organizations and preferred provider organizations, had been introduced to compete against the more traditional pattern of fee-for-service treatments backed by private health insurance.

The results of these changes could not be applied directly to the United Kingdom in predicting the effects of a more competitive NHS, and in any case the results themselves were mixed; but many of the negative ones were used to cast doubt upon the wisdom of moving the NHS farther along the competitive road.[4] Much was made of the fact that a central aim of the American changes had failed to materialize: far from being contained, costs had continued to increase, sucking a swelling proportion of the national wealth into health care.[5] In order to sharpen their competitiveness and to offer more choice to patients, hospitals had had to invest in up-to-date equipment which had not only been costly in itself but had often led to a duplication of services in areas where several hospitals were competing against each other for the custom of a finite population. Equipment had often lain idle and staff been underemployed as hospitals had striven towards individual self-sufficiency in the market rather than complementary collaboration within a planned network of services. The high transaction costs of actually running the market, such as those of advertising, marketing and invoicing, had exerted further inflationary pressures on spending. There were, as expected, some beneficial results in all of this: competition had pivoted around the quality as much as the cost of what was provided, and patients had enjoyed more choice of treatment. Yet the continual pressure on providers to control their costs had led also to less welcome outcomes in the wake of the price regulations that were introduced. Profit margins had fallen, some hospitals had been forced to close, and others had rationalized their product ranges to gain the benefits of specialization. The scope for cross-subsidization within hospitals, whereby less profitable procedures or poorer patients were compensated by the income from profitable treatments and richer patients, had diminished, causing effort to be concentrated on the more lucrative forms of care and patients of uncertain financial status to be excluded or 'dumped' on public hospitals.

The application of these American experiences to the NHS, hazardous under any circumstances but particularly so in the politically emotive atmosphere of the debate, was done in a way that enabled the critics of the White Paper both to have their cake and eat it. On the one hand, fears were expressed that the worst aspects of the American experience would become manifest in the internal market of the NHS: hospitals would pursue their self-interests with scant regard to community needs, profitable services would take precedence over needed ones, inefficient hospitals would close, transaction costs would soar, and the selective admission of patients on financial grounds would become commonplace. On the other hand, it was thought that the internal market would embody so many idiosyncratic peculiarities that the beneficial effects of competition, such as they were, would not be felt. The inability of the British system to price its services or measure their quality would make a mockery of the notion of consumer sovereignty; the inevitable conflict of interests between health authorities as purchasers and as providers would frustrate the principle of open competition; the exclusion of patients from the internal market would certainly not enhance (and would probably constrict) their scope for choice; and the exclusion of contractual disputations from judicial determination would shield defaulters behind the cloak of political or bureaucratic expediency.

The second theme in the symphony of protest was that, whatever might be the principled merits or otherwise of market competition in the NHS, the particular form of the market envisaged in *Working for Patients* would be unworkable in practice. There were many strands to the argument, only the bare essences of which can be captured in a few paragraphs. They centred upon the viability of the district health authorities as commissioners, of the general practitioners as budget holders, and of the hospitals as self-governing trusts.

First of all, major and possibly insurmountable difficulties were foreseen for the DHAs in managing the divorce between their functions as commissioners and as providers.[6] The principle of the separation of functions was one of the central features of *Working for Patients* that had commanded early and quite widespread approval. Hitherto, health authorities had often had difficulty in balancing the needs and interests of their resident populations against the needs and interests of the hospitals and other provider units that happened to be located within their boundaries and for which they were therefore managerially responsible; but they had begun to take steps to address the problem. Even before the publication of the White Paper, changes in the management structures within the DHAs had begun to effect a separation of functions by bolstering the status and authority of the unit general managers (on the provider side) and distancing them from their bosses, the district general managers (DGMs). In this sense the White Paper could be viewed as an extension and formalization of the creative tension already existing within the local management structures.

With the passage of time, however, the practical difficulties of effecting a complete separation became increasingly apparent, for however much autonomy was granted in principle to the hospitals and other units providing the care, the awkward fact remained that they had no independent legal authority to enter into any kind of contractual arrangement. Unless they opted for trust status, hospitals and other units would remain under the management control of their parent authority, and it was only that authority which could commit them contractually. The rather confusing prospect therefore began to form of hospitals and other units entering into trading relationships with the very authorities to which they were managerially accountable. For their part, the authorities and their senior officers were in a similarly ambiguous position: as the commissioning agencies, they would be expected to strike the best possible deals with their chosen providers (some of whom would be their own directly managed units), while as the managers of the provider units they would be expected to negotiate the best possible terms with their commissioning authorities.

The DGMs, as the senior managers responsible for both commissioning and providing, were caught distinctly in the spotlight of this dilemma.[7] Understandably unwilling to commit themselves to one side or the other of the widening divide until they could clearly foresee where their best interests lay, they found themselves resorting to various expediencies to maintain their credibility and minimize their conflicting responsibilities. Some found refuge in the notion of the Chinese wall, helpfully suggested by the NHS Management Executive as an aid to resolving any crisis of identity that might be felt.[8] Though never explicitly defined, a Chinese wall was, by implication, an invisible yet impermeable barrier constructed in the minds of authority members and senior managers preventing them from knowing anything about their responsibilities as providers when managing the commissioning function, and anything about their roles as commissioners when acting as providers.

Alternative and ultimately more feasible solutions lay in structural change within the districts.[9] In the long term, as ministers were quick to point out, the problem would gradually resolve itself as the number of self-governing trusts increased and the separation of functions became absolute.[10] In the medium term, the problem could be eased by the creation of new commissioning authorities, possibly formed through the amalgamation of two or more DHAs, that would have to remain technically accountable to the parent authorities until new legislation could be passed conferring a legally autonomous status upon them, but that would function to all intents and purposes independently of them. In the short term, various models of district organization were suggested that would minimize the scope for ambiguity in the roles of senior managers. Based upon the experiences of some authorities (such as those in East Anglia) already operating a kind of internal market, some models saw the DGM as heading up the purchasing function only, leaving the unit general managers directly accountable to the health authority; others envisaged the DGM as co-ordinating the provider units, leaving the commissioning teams as directly accountable; and others regarded the DGM as a neutral broker, mediating between the commissioning and providing functions on the authority's behalf.[11] Each model raised questions (albeit differing ones) of feasibility, and each implied an organizational turbulence that would need to be added to the scales in judging the balance of advantage in forging the internal market.

If the anticipated structural difficulties facing the DHAs in coping with the separation of functions were great, those of actually making the commissioning process work were seen eventually to be even more severe. Much of the early debate on the White Paper had surrounded the controversial (and therefore newsworthy) proposals for budget-holding general practices and self-governing hospital trusts. The demands that were facing the DHAs in their new commissioning roles went largely unrecognized and unremarked for many months, not least because of the scant attention they received in the White Paper itself. By the beginning of 1990, however, doubts were beginning to surface about the capacity of the health authorities to execute the commissioning process as its component parts became more clear.

A key step in the process, requiring the authorities to measure the needs of their resident populations for health and medical care and to prioritize them in a way that would inform their purchasing strategies, was not intrinsically new, for DHAs had always supposedly based their policies upon their assessments of local needs. Yet the conceptual and procedural difficulties in doing so had invariably impaired their capacity to plan the development of their services in such an ideal fashion. The very notion of need had proved notoriously difficult to define in ways that could be used in the planning process, and the prospect of arranging a heterogeneous array of needs into an explicit hierarchy of importance for the purpose of deciding service priorities had usually been too daunting even to contemplate. In consequence, local judgements about priorities among differing kinds of needs were usually revealed only implicitly in the ways the money was spent, not in separately articulated statements of policy intent. The internal market, however, would require priority-setting to become both more explicit and more visible: not only would the health authorities have to determine their priorities for care with greater transparency than they had been accustomed to doing in the past, but also the steady rise in the number of trusts would heighten the public visibility of the process of needs assessment and service planning as it became increasingly the core remaining function of the DHAs. Whether they could rise adequately to the challenge became a matter of fascinated speculation.

Even if this particular obstacle could be surmounted with reasonable success, there remained the further task of translating the local assessments of needs into purchasing requirements that were capable of expression in contractual terms. This task, like that of the assessment of local needs, was not entirely new, since something like it had in principle guided the allocation of management budgets to hospitals and units under the existing system. But the introduction of explicitly formulated contracts, in many ways the linchpin of the commissioning process, forced into the open a number of practical and intellectual difficulties that had not hitherto been faced in quite such a transparent way.[8] Foremost among them were the issues of price and quality.[12] It was doubted, for example, whether the prices to be specified in the contracts could be determined with the level of discrimination necessary for the market to do its job.[13] It was recognized that prices had to be related to the costs incurred by providers, including any charges payable on their capital assets, and that these would be highly variable among providers. It was recognized, too, that in the formative stages of the market the prices would have to be such as to sustain the existing flow of resources since staff, buildings and equipment could not substantially be altered in a short space of time. But if the market were to generate the expected efficiencies in the production of care in the longer term and to ensure that resources flowed in greater quantity towards the more efficient producers, price competition would have to occur eventually, and providers would have to find realistic ways of pricing their wares.

This was, however, a matter in which experience and precedence had little to offer. Existing trading agreements between health authorities had been based upon prices that often reflected nothing more than the outcome of bilateral negotiations between the two parties,[14] and the Resource Management Initiative, which was widely regarded as the major forum in which managers were learning the art of pricing their services, was failing to make the progress in the theory and practice of pricing that many were expecting.[15] As if to anticipate and forestall such problems, the government and its supporters argued from an early stage in the debate that a sophisticated means of fixing prices was unnecessary, and even that a standard schedule of prices would suffice to begin with.[16] By the end of 1989 the talk from Whitehall was of a national price tariff with possible local variations (and therefore price competition) only at the margins.[17] The result, as a leading health economist pointed out, was that procedural feasibility had been secured at the expense of radical change, for 'without price flexibility there are no financial signals in the marketplace to show which hospitals are efficient and which could be better managed'.[18]

Price determination was not the only rock of viability upon which it was feared the commissioning process might founder: it was also doubted whether the quality of many forms of care could be described and measured with the precision required of a contractual agreement between a purchaser and a provider. There were close parallels with the problem of price determination: it needed to be done if buyers in the market were to be able to make informed choices among competing providers and to be satisfied that they had got value for their money, but little useful progress had been made in developing ways of measuring the quality of the care that patients received, particularly in terms of their subsequent improvements in health.[19] Nevertheless, experience had been gained with other ways of measuring quality, and what was perceived initially as a problem came to be seen as an opportunity for a major and long-overdue investment in methods of specifying and monitoring the quality of the care given by hospitals and other providers.[20] By the beginning of 1990, in a Departmental document on contracting for clinical care, model contracts were being produced with quality measurements of ambitious complexity, many of which would have been all but impossible to monitor.[21] Reality in the initial stages was inevitably more prosaic: health authorities had little previous experience of defining quality in contractual terms, and the first contracts that were drawn up between the health authorities and their providers generally lacked a rigorous approach to the specification of quality, especially in relation to health outcomes.[22]

The threat that might be posed to the viability of the internal market by the failure of the health authorities to develop their roles as commissioners was that of its domination by the provider hospitals. It was seen as essential to the success of the market that the health authorities as purchasing agencies should rapidly acquire the confidence, skills and authority to hold their own in their negotiations with the providers; yet the fear was commonly expressed that the providers would come to dominate the relationship, resulting in the provision of services that it was in their own interests to supply rather than services that the purchasers wished to have.[23] Initially, at least, the power and the experience would be on the side of the providers, particularly the large and prestigious acute hospitals, and so, too, would the managerial expertise if many senior managers saw their future interests as lying on the provider rather than the purchaser side of the market. Even though the health authorities would receive the financial resources and would in principle have the power to disburse them as they wished, their independence in spending them might be compromised by the ability of the large providers to forestall any widespread changes in service provision. That such concerns might have been well grounded became apparent in May 1990 with the resignation of the DGM of a prominent London authority, reportedly on the grounds of disillusionment at the ascendancy that the London teaching hospitals were thought to be gaining over the commissioning authorities in the capital.[24]

If a weight of sceptical and hostile opinion surrounded the feasibility of the split between the purchasing and providing functions of the DHAs, no less an amount was attracted to the White Paper's proposals for general practice, especially the notion of GPs holding their own budgets from which to purchase care for their patients. Even the principle of the scheme was seen to be of dubious viability: prior to the publication of the White Paper two leading commentators had warned that the spirit of free enterprise was alien to the culture of many doctors and would not be acceptable to them.[25] As if to demonstrate the force of that prediction, GPs in Powys decided, shortly before the White Paper's publication, to shun a local pilot budget-holding scheme.[26] Even Professor Enthoven, widely regarded as the consultant architect to the market's design, expressed his doubts about the idea, suggesting that, prior to their widespread introduction, practice budgets might be suitable for testing through a demonstration project.[27]

A major element of concern over the viability of the scheme was the size of the budget. The White Paper had proposed that practices with more than 11,000 registered patients (later reduced to 9,000) should be eligible to apply for budgets, their illustrative value being between £600,000 and £700,000. Not only was this regarded as an intrinsically small amount to cover the costs that would be charged against it,[28] but it was also widely perceived as too small to cope with the yearly variations that would be bound to occur in the incidence of costly events.[29] A small deviation in the annual pattern of expensive illnesses (except those costing in excess of £5,000, for which the excess costs would be borne by the health authority) might break the budget. Professor Enthoven himself suggested later that a practice size of 100,000 patients would be needed to spread the risks adequately from year to year.[30] In the absence of larger budgets, it was feared that GPs might actively select or cull their patients with a bias towards the fit and the healthy,[31] that they would come under pressure from insurance companies to encourage their patients to take out personal private policies,[32] and that they would be pestered by patients seeking to supplement the practice budget from their private resources in order to secure a treatment that might not otherwise be offered.

Not only was it questioned whether the budgets could be made to work acceptably, but also the capacity of the doctors themselves as business managers came into question. Holding a budget would be time-consuming and difficult, requiring doctors to develop new skills and abilities: formulating a purchasing strategy, negotiating with the provider hospitals, handling the administrative and accounting elements of the contract, and monitoring expenditure against the budget. It was plain that, at least to start with, budget-holding practices would receive considerable advice and assistance from the regional health authorities, but the demands upon the practices themselves remained considerable. A survey of GPs in Merseyside, conducted before the publication of *Working for Patients*, signalled the extent of the changes required.[33] Fewer than half of the 450 GPs in the survey held practice management meetings, almost three-quarters had no computer in the practice, and half reported difficulties in the management of innovation. The survey's authors concluded that, while it did not reveal the doctors as incompetent managers, it did 'demonstrate a basic lack of readiness to take on the managerial challenges before them, even assuming control of practice budgets'.

Many other difficulties and drawbacks were foreseen in the actual operation of practice budgets: their administration would be costly in time and money, they would impede the free flow of patients within and between hospitals following an initial consultation with the hospital doctor, they would effectively impose cash limits on the clinical care provided by GPs that could subsequently be varied according to political will, and they would contain inadequate incentives to doctors to participate in the scheme. A particular difficulty, to which both GPs[34] and consultants[35] drew attention, concerned the nature of what it was that the GPs would be buying from the provider hospitals. The Working Paper on practice budgets had specified 37 surgical procedures that would be chargeable against the budgets, but it was argued that GPs rarely requested particular operations. They would not, for example, usually request a hysterectomy: rather, they would refer women for consultant opinion with symptoms that might or might not result in that procedure. The difficulty that this would cause for the management of the practice budget (that the practice would rarely know in advance the full cost of any referral) would be minimized in a block contract (which would give the practice access to a defined range of facilities without regard to the particular procedures or treatments carried out), but would be accentuated in the cost-and-volume and cost-per-case contracts which practices were expected increasingly to adopt.

The relationship between the purchasing strategies of the budget-holding practices and of the DHAs became a further source of concern: the capacity of these practices to impair the commissioning responsibilities of the DHAs would, it was feared, become increasingly damaging as the number of budget-holding practices grew.[36] In part this was because the element of each practice budget allowed for the purchase of hospital care would be deducted from the financial allocations to the DHAs, thereby progressively depleting the volume of resources the authorities would have at their disposal. Not only would this diminish the scale of the districts' commissioning activities, but it would also threaten the goal of a synoptic district-wide approach to the planning and provision of services. For however carefully a DHA might gauge its population's needs and plan its service requirements accordingly, the budget-holding practices within its boundaries might well pursue their own eccentric buying policies, without regard to their complementarity with the district strategy. Indeed, it was seen to be of the essence of the budget-holding scheme that these practices *should* pursue the best interests of their own patients, at odds if necessary with the district strategy, for there would otherwise be little purpose in having separate budgets. A commonly paraded benefit of budget-holding was that, by allowing individual practices to purchase different and better services for their own patients, a salutary pressure would be exerted upon the commissioning authorities to do likewise. Any such benefit would evaporate if the budget-holding practices meekly conformed with the district's purchasing strategy.

While most of the critical attention to general practice was focused upon the White Paper's innovative proposals for budget-holding practices, the other practices that would not hold their own budgets were also seen increasingly as a threat to the viability of the market, for the freedom of these doctors to refer their patients to the consultants of their choice (long regarded as a central bulwark of their clinical freedom) could plainly come into conflict with the contracts being placed by the DHAs. If the GPs in these practices retained their customary freedom to refer their patients wherever they wished, then the commissioning authorities would have to compromise their free choice of providers and place their contracts with the hospitals selected by the referring doctors. If, on the other hand, the commissioners were allowed to place their contracts entirely with the providers of their choice, then the doctors would have to limit the bulk of their referrals to the contracted hospitals, whether they liked it or not, for otherwise the hospitals would receive no reimbursement for the care they provided. One way or the other, something would have to give.

The problem, and a possible solution, had been recognized by Professor Enthoven in his 1985 monograph.[37] If the DHAs were to maximize the efficiency of their purchasing decisions, he argued, they would need to restrict the referrals of the GPs to those hospitals with which they had contracted. To endow them with the authority to do so, he suggested that it should be they (rather than the family practitioner committees) that held the GPs' contracts. *Working for Patients*, however, proposed no such change to the GPs' contract, suggesting instead a number of other ways in which the potential conflict could be managed. In particular, it highlighted the importance of a tight collusion between a DHA and its GPs in compiling the district's portfolio of contracts, and it stressed the need for each DHA to retain a portion of its budget to cover the costs, on a case-by-case basis, of essential referrals to hospitals for which no contractual cover existed.

The potency of the threat posed to the freedom of the GPs in the non budget-holding practices by the logic of the commissioning role assigned to the DHAs formed a central motif in the fabric of medical opposition, eliciting elaborate linguistic attempts from the Department of Health to face both ways at once. A discussion document from the Management Executive in September 1989 declared the Department's objective as that of 'securing the referral patterns which local GPs wish to see put in place unless there are compelling reasons for not doing so'.[38] The document went on to note, with studied understatement, that the requirements of the GPs and of the DHAs 'will not always match', and that 'careful consultation will be important to align the aspirations of the GPs with the plans of the DHAs for contract placement, and to secure the best balance of advantage'. That the difficulties in doing so would be considerable were highlighted in the early experiences emerging in 1990 from a prototype internal market established in the South Western region. According to one report, two contiguous districts within the region had negotiated the transfer of 36 general medical beds from one district to the other, together with the appropriate financial wherewithal, and had expected the referrals from local GPs to accord with the arrangement.[39] That this expectation was not met gave rise to confrontation between the districts over the financial responsibility for the treatment of patients referred outwith the arrangement and for whom no contractual provisions had been made. 'Purchasers have to make clear to their GPs the services they are or are not buying on their behalf', the financial director of one district was reported as saying – an imperative that sat rather uncomfortably with an earlier assurance from the Department of Health that all GPs would be free to refer outwith their authorities' contractual frameworks.

The White Paper's proposals for self-governing hospital trusts formed a third main focus of doubt about the practicability of the market it was proposing. Many of the doubts surrounded the ability of the trusts to manage their affairs as commercially autonomous hospitals in a competitive market.[40] They would have had little experience in business planning, marketing, pricing and billing, and it was clear that they would need to undergo a great deal of corporate learning to enable them to acquire the requisite skills in a short space of time. They would also need to find ways of reconciling the clinical autonomy of the consultants with the market imperative of financial viability. A tension between the interests of the doctors and the solvency of the hospitals had always existed and had never been resolved satisfactorily: under the existing system of management budgets it had always been possible for consultants to create a financial deficit by doing more work than the hospital's budget permitted, causing many DHAs to incur greater financial commitments than their revenue allocations allowed. Ward closures and deferred payments to creditors in the latter months of the financial year had been used increasingly throughout the 1980s as devices for coping with such problems, but these might stand revealed as inadequate in the internal market if they caused the rupture of contractual obligations. The new consultant contract proposed in *Working for Patients* was designed in part to constrain the clinical autonomy of the doctors within the structures of the business plans, as also were the emerging systems (most notably resource management) for the more intimate involvement of clinicians in the management of their hospitals. In the longer term, the freedom bestowed upon the trusts to employ their own clinical staff on their own terms and conditions would give them a further potent weapon to ensure compliance. Yet doubts were inevitably raised, in view of the medical profession's demonstrable capacity to preserve its own freedoms, about the viability of such devices to secure their objectives.

Further and widespread misgivings were aired about the practicability of the scheme proposed in *Working for Patients* for charging all NHS hospitals (whether trusts or directly managed hospitals) for the value of their capital assets. The principle of capital charging was sound: if there was to be fair competition between NHS and independent hospitals, the former would have to submit to the same financial disciplines as the latter. They could no longer enjoy the use of capital as a free good. Yet because of the totally innovative nature of capital charging in the NHS, its feasibility was uncertain, notwithstanding the publication of two working papers on the matter.[41] How would the capital assets of the hospitals be valued for determining the basis of their charges? Would the site value of a hospital be based upon its current use as a hospital or its potential use for other purposes? How should a hospital's originating debt be divided between the loan element (on which interest would be payable) and the capital element (on which a public dividend might be levied)? How would the interest rate and the dividend levels be determined to ensure a level playing field between the public and private sectors? How should the money levied through the charges be recycled into the NHS?

To these questions of viability, for which precedence offered few solutions, the teaching hospitals (especially those in London) added further ones of self-interest.[42] The high value of hospital sites in London and other large cities could, it was feared, give rise to capital charges of a magnitude that would render the hospitals entirely uncompetitive. The second working paper on capital charging, published in the summer of 1989, failed to allay the concern. It confirmed that hospitals would be required to pay their charges in the form of annual deposits (rather than as single once-and-for-all payments), and that the money would be recycled into the NHS as yearly allocations to the DHAs as compensation for the higher prices they would be charged by the hospitals. Provided each DHA placed all its contracts with its 'own' hospitals, the flow of money would be cyclical within a closed system: each authority would, in effect, receive back the capital charges that had been levied on the hospitals within its boundary, thereby ensuring that those hospitals continued to be funded at the same level as before.[43] It was, however, of the essence of the internal market that closed systems should be broken open and that DHAs should, with time, place their contracts more widely, to include independent hospitals or NHS hospitals in other districts offering better value for money. The threatening possibility thus arose of DHAs in London and other large cities receiving yearly allocations that reflected the capital charges levied on the hospitals within their boundaries, but placing their contracts elsewhere, where hospitals with lower asset valuations could afford to charge lower prices. The scene appeared to be set for a potentially bruising conflict between market imperatives and political expediency: either the market would be allowed to work against the high-cost hospitals, causing them to dismantle their beds, lay off their staff or reduce their services, or the political price to be paid for such a highly visible contraction of well-known hospitals would be judged to be too high, and the natural outworkings of the market would be frustrated through some form of bureaucratic intervention.

There were, then, many expressed fears that the particular form of the market envisaged in *Working for Patients* would contain so many problems and difficulties as to be all but unworkable. In the early months of 1989 a deeply veined scepticism was evident that the internal market would ever materialize in anything like the form envisaged in the White Paper. With the unpeeling of each new layer of implication, the feasibility of the market's unmodified implementation appeared to recede. As the year progressed, however, and the government's implacable determination to press ahead became ever more apparent, the symphony of protest moved on to another theme and a different key: the argument that the market would prove unworkable gave way to the claim that, even if it were technically feasible, it was structured in a way that would frustrate the achievement of its own objectives. The dominant issues here were those of choice, accessibility and competition.

The White Paper and subsequent ministerial apologetics laid much emphasis on the theme of choice: it was said that patients in the current dispensation often had little if any choice over the time or place at which they received their treatment, and it was promised that the deficit would be rectified in the new order of things. Yet the internal market of *Working for Patients* seemed to be structured in a way that would inhibit any such beneficial change. The general theory of markets endows consumers with choice because of their participation as buyers: if they do not like what is on offer at one place, they have the choice of taking their custom elsewhere. The market proposed in *Working for Patients*, however, embodied the particular characteristic of excluding from its dealings those who would consume its products. It would not be the patients themselves who would be shopping around in the market for the best deals, it would be surrogate buyers doing it on their behalf. At best, patients would merely have the choice between one of two surrogate buyers – a budget-holding general practice or the DHA. At worst, if no budget-holding practice existed in their locality, patients would be denied even this limited choice: they would have no option but to conform with the contracts placed by the authority. Those who do not pay the piper must make do with the tunes that are played for them.

The apparent gulf between the White Paper's rhetoric of greater patient choice and the impending reality provided a focal point of disillusionment for groups across a range of political opinion. It disappointed those to the right of the spectrum, who had hoped that the review would take the opportunity of opening the NHS up to commercial access by individual patients as paying customers.[44] It alarmed a clutch of patients' organizations, concerned that people might be required to travel excessive distances to receive treatment, with no alternative choice of a local provider.[45] And it formed a central strand in the fabric of medical opposition to the White Paper.[46] Opinion, however, was not unanimous: the Director of the

National Association of Health Authorities was reported as discerning 'whole areas of greater patient choice' in the White Paper,[47] and others pointed out not only that an extensive choice for most patients was illusory even under the existing scheme of things, but that choice may not be a highly valued quality in any case. Most patients, the argument ran, are more concerned with securing good treatment in quick time than with choosing the location of their care or the doctor providing it. If the market could sharpen up the quality and timing of care, the issue of choice would lose its potency.

Whether the internal market could deliver its promise to improve the accessibility of care became a further source of scepticism, however. It pivoted around the White Paper's specific and explicit promise of reductions in waiting times for hospital admission – an indicator that, probably because of its relative ease of measurement and its obvious relevance to people's needs, had for long been regarded as a sensitive token of the well-being of the NHS. For the White Paper to offer such an explicit hostage to the future may have been unavoidable in the light of the government's need to convince the people of the tangible benefits to be had from the reforms. That it was also a calculated risk, however, was apparent from the lack of any theoretical analysis of how the market would benignly affect the size of waiting lists. The extensively progressive stratagems of efficiency savings and cost improvement programmes that the government had deployed throughout the 1980s had failed to produce many widespread or sustainable reductions in waiting times in many parts of the UK, and the government's dedicated attack on waiting lists had yet to yield demonstrably good results.[48] That the internal market would succeed where these other initiatives had largely failed was, in the view of some experts (including the government's special adviser on waiting lists), too much to expect.[49]

The theory, by implication, was that geographical mismatches existed between the demand for, and the availability of, hospital surgical resources that could be corrected by allowing DHAs and budget-holding general practices to shop around for places where waiting times were short or capacity was spare. Further pressure could be exerted on the hospitals to reduce their waiting times by specifying maximum acceptable times within the terms of the contracts placed with them.[50] The reality, it was feared, would not be quite so simple: waiting lists were thought by many to be highest in areas and in specialties which were underfunded or in which the consultants were engaged extensively in private work, and the obvious point was made that a contract cannot exist for something that is simply unattainable.[51] It was recognized that it would be possible in the short term for some purchasers to secure a faster access to surgical services than would otherwise be the case (if that is how they chose to spend their money), and it was thought that the budget-holding general practices, in particular, might find it attractive to use their resources to clear their backlogs of patients awaiting elective surgery. Yet preferential treatment for the patients of budget-holding practices could, in the long run, be secured only at the expense of an increase in waiting times for other patients unless a growth occurred in the total output of surgical services. To conceal an overall insufficiency of services (if that indeed was what was underlying the stubbornly large waiting lists) by redistributing it from one locality to another, or from one group of patients to another, was not regarded as an adequate long-term solution.

Nor was the prospect of patients shuttling around the country in search of the shortest waiting times regarded as terribly realistic. That there should be some element of travel from one district to another was an essential feature of the internal market, for without such travel little scope would exist for purchasers to move beyond their traditional suppliers. If ministerial visions were to materialize of money following patients to the most efficient providers, the patients would have to move in the first place. Yet their opportunity for doing so, as the Department of Health itself conceded in a 1989 discussion document, would be geographically patterned.[12] Those living in conurbations and other densely populated territories might indeed enjoy access to a range of hospitals and other units within reasonable travelling distance, but patients in predominantly rural settings would have little such choice, continuing to be dependent upon the single hospital from which they had always received their care. Indeed, the charge was heard that *Working for Patients* was largely the product of London-based politicians, reflecting the distinctive problems of health-care provision in South-East England, with little real relevance to many other parts of the UK. The sheer difficulties that many patients would experience in travelling long distances for care would, it was claimed, impair the objective of linking excess demand with spare capacity.[52]

The emphasis given to the claim was somewhat muted in the early months of the debate when the market was seen as being restricted to elective surgical care and many patients were thought likely to be willing to suffer the burdens and costs of travelling considerable distances for the speedier treatment of their less urgent complaints.[53] Indeed, there was empirical support for Professor Enthoven's view that 'if it means having your operation done promptly by very skilled people, then it may be a small price to pay to have to travel'.[27] However, with the growing realization that the commissioning process would extend beyond the limited confines of elective surgery to embrace the total spectrum of health-care provision,[54] doubts increased about the capacity of the wider market to fulfil the objectives held out for it. The impracticability of people travelling much beyond the boundaries of their home districts for all sorts of services seemed to scupper the prospects of greater efficiency through the discriminating placement of contracts.

The likely difficulties that purchasers would experience in gaining access to multiple providers were not the only grounds for doubting the market's claim to sharpen efficiency through competition. The nature of the contractual relation between purchasers and providers would, it was claimed, further inhibit the fruitful flowering of the competitive ethos. Initially, at least, most contracts would be of the simple block variety, not least because of the time-lag required to develop the costing and information systems needed to support a more sophisticated type of relationship. Yet the very nature of block contracts, allowing an unspecified number of patients access to an agreed range of facilities in return for a global fee, was scarcely the discriminating tool that conventional markets were accustomed to using. Not only would it limit the obligations of the provider hospitals simply to the supply of a set of facilities rather than the delivery of specified services, but it would also tend to relegate price competition to the margins of a provider's activities where capacity was spare or an end-of-year surplus became unexpectedly available.[51] Moreover, the sheer size of the block contracts that DHAs were expected to place in the early years of the internal market would, it was feared, make life difficult for the small purchasers and the small providers who were supposed to constitute the market's competitive spice. On the purchasing side, the budget-holding general practices, commanding far fewer resources than the bulk-buying DHAs, might have difficulty in getting the hospitals to tender for the small volume of services they would be seeking to buy;[55] and on the provider side of the market, it was feared that smaller independent hospitals would be forced out of the competition by the bigger trusts and directly managed hospitals able to quote favourable prices for large orders.[56]

The natural tendency for oligopolies to form in a market dominated by block contracts might, moreover, be unnaturally enhanced by the anti-competitive behaviour of the providers themselves. Competition is not the inevitable consequence of a market environment: providers might seek to preserve their interests just as much by collaborating with each other as by engaging in competition. The theory of markets suggests that the threat of competition should be sufficient to curb any such nascent tendencies towards conspiratorial behaviour on the part of the sellers, but it was feared that the new internal market in the NHS would, at least initially, contain so many uncertainties and instabilities that the providers who were supposed to be in a competitive relationship might choose instead to prevent the risk of chaos and collapse by sharing out the market among themselves.[57] Independent hospitals, in particular, might (it was suggested) find this an attractive option, for while the White Paper offered rich pickings for the independent sector in the long term, it posed threats of viability in the short term as the private sector reorganized itself to accommodate the new competition from the trust and directly managed hospitals.[58] It was thought possible that the independent sector might respond by seeking to convince the DHAs (as the main purchasers) that their requirements could best be met not by obliging the private hospitals to compete with the NHS for custom, but by extending the kinds of joint collaborative scheme that had been developing for some time and that (as shown in Chapter 2) had provided one of the foundations of experience upon which the White Paper was built. Indeed, it was even argued that, in the short run, such behaviour might be positively commendable to prevent any unforeseen disasters from occurring in the early months and years;[57] but whether the formation of such cartels would be acceptable in the long run to the Audit Commission, the Department of Trade and Industry and the Office of Fair Trading was less certain.

There were, then, various doubts about the capacity of the internal market, even if it could be made to work in the form envisaged in *Working for Patients*, to achieve some of the key objectives that were set for it. The fourth and final theme in the symphony of protest had a similarly negative refrain: that the market would damage or even destroy many of the best features of the NHS. The dominant issues here were those of cost, co-ordination, equality, democracy and medical trust.

The capacity of the NHS to control its costs (particularly its administrative costs) had for long been regarded as one of its strengths. Indeed, a number of structural features of the service had repeatedly commended themselves to outside observers for their beneficially deflationary pressures on costs with no discernibly deleterious effects on the health of the people. The cost of raising the revenue for the NHS is low, being effectively borne by the Inland Revenue; the cost of administering the service is low because of the absence of most of the transaction expenditures involved in running a market; and salary levels in the NHS are low, relative to those in many other countries, because of the position of the NHS as virtually the sole purchaser of medical, nursing and other technical skills. In consequence, a persistently lower proportion of the gross national product of the United Kingdom than of most other industrialized countries has been spent on health and medical care, and, within that total, a distinctively lower proportion has been consumed by managerial and administrative functions. Cross-national comparisons in patterns of expenditure are notoriously unreliable but, for what it is worth, the figure has frequently been quoted that administrative costs in the NHS amount to some 5 per cent of the total expenditure, compared to 20 per cent or more under various insurance plans in the USA.[59]

While the implementation of *Working for Patients* would change neither the capacity of government to impose cash limits on the total resources available to the NHS nor the cheapness of the means by which they were raised, the introduction of the internal market would, it was argued, remove other restraining pressures on costs. Persistent and widespread fears were expressed of an escalation of administrative and managerial expenses which, unless adequately compensated, would inevitably attract resources away from the care of patients. Such fears were not unfounded: the potential complexity and cost of operating the internal market, veiled in the White Paper itself, was revealed in all its nightmarish detail in a draft document from the Department of Health in December 1989 which itemized the Byzantine systems of record-keeping, billing and accounting that would be needed to ensure the market could work.[60]

The numbers and cost of the additional managerial, financial and administrative staff needed to operate the new systems of the internal market became a matter of intense speculation. Mr Clarke, in evidence to the House of Commons Social Services Committee, declined to suggest a figure,[61] but others willingly did it for him. Estimates of the numbers of extra accountants required to work the system ranged from 250 by the Audit Commission[57] to 1,000 by the Healthcare Financial Management Association (of whom 600 would be working on capital charging).[41] The cost of employing them was estimated to be as much as £25 million. The total cost to the government of implementing the White Paper between the date of its publication and the date of its coming into force was predicted early in 1989 to be of the order of £500 million, a forecast that proved to be remarkably accurate. By the end of 1989 the government had provided an additional £85 million for the NHS in England to fund the work on the implementation of the White Paper, and it anticipated the allocation of a further £300 million in the financial year 1990–1.[62] Including an additional £165 million for setting up the information systems required to make the market operational by 1991, the government's own estimate of the global cost of implementing *Working for Patients* was therefore of the order of £550 million. The recurrent cost of actually running the market in a full year was estimated in the National Health Service and Community Care Bill, presented in Parliament in November 1989, to be about £217 million at 1989 prices, of which the major portion (£155 million) would be swallowed up by increased managerial expenditures. Harking back to the dominant refrain of the White Paper, however, the Bill was quick to point out that these additional costs would be outweighed by 'improvements in the operation of services, which will create more opportunities for achieving value for money from the resources employed'. The veracity of that asseveration was, of course, at the heart of the concern about the supposedly high transaction costs of the internal market.

It was not only administrative costs that were feared set to surge in the new dispensation: inflationary pressures were also foreseen in other areas, most notably the salaries of doctors and other clinical staff with skills in high demand. The nub of the problem was seen to lie in the freedoms that the self-governing hospital trusts would have to employ the staff they required (including consultant medical staff) on whatever terms and conditions they could negotiate. The effect would be to replace a single monopsonistic purchaser of labour (the NHS) with many purchasers (the trust and independent hospitals) while retaining a single monopolistic supplier (in the case of doctors, the General Medical Council through its monopoly control over their registration).[63] The consequence might be an escalation in wages and salaries as hospitals were set in competition with each other for the employment of people with rare or specialist skills. The additional prospect of an end to the uniform, national contract for hospital consultants, likely to lead eventually to the redundancy of the Review Body on Doctors' and Dentists' Remuneration, would merely hasten the demise of nationally negotiated salaries and usher in an era of salary inflation as the autonomous hospitals fought to preserve their market competitiveness by attracting the most able staff. Eventually, it was even suggested, doctors might emulate footballers in being the subject of transfer fees from one hospital to another, reflecting the value they commanded in the market.[64]

The threat that the internal market might pose to the planned development and co-ordination of services, long regarded as a distinctive strength of a nationally based health service, generated further alarm. Though the reality of co-ordinated care had always been less rosy than the promise, the NHS was founded upon the principle of a planned and complementary system of care offering a broadly comparable service in all parts of the country, in principle comprehensive in scope, and with a minimum of duplication or overlap. The great structural reforms of 1974 and, to a lesser extent, of 1982 had been designed in part to strengthen the integration of the different elements of the system and to facilitate its strategic planning. Yet many of the key features of the internal market would, it was feared, deliberately undermine the historical commitment to a nationally planned service.[65] The failure of *Working for Patients* to integrate its proposals into the government's plans for the future of community care and its promise of an end to national wage and salary structures were two of the sources of disquiet, but others also surfaced in this context. The existence of multiple buyers in those districts which contained several budget-holding general practices would necessarily militate against a comprehensive purchasing strategy.[36] The transformation of hospitals and community units into self-governing trusts would replace networks of interlocking services with autonomous outlets intent on pursuing their own interests in the market. The closure of beds, wards and even hospitals would be dictated largely by the outworkings of the market, whatever their impact upon local service structures. And the hospitals would have a direct incentive to develop and market the services that were most likely to ensure their prosperity in preference to those that would contribute to the needs and requirements of a locality. As the *Financial Times* put it, 'out goes planning and rationing by managers and doctors; in comes competition and the price mechanism'.[66]

The issue of the local provision of essential services became a specific and emotive focus of the generalized concern about the market's capacity to fragment the planned provision of a balanced range of services. The White Paper enunciated as a precondition of a hospital's bid for trust status that it should provide essential core services to its local population, including accident and emergency facilities, where no alternative provision existed. The subsequent working paper on self-governing hospitals decreed the definition of a core service to be a matter for the DHA to determine, not the Department of Health, although Mr Clarke was careful to emphasize that DHAs would have a statutory duty to continue to make a comprehensive range of services available to their resident populations.[67] The fear persisted, however, that the financial pressures upon the hospital trusts to dispense with commercially unattractive services, however greatly they may be needed locally, and to gain the beneficial effects of scale through greater specialization, would negate the policy of meeting the full range of people's needs through the local district general hospital. Such fears were not eased by the reported minute of a meeting in 1989 between the senior doctors of a London teaching hospital and an official of the Department of Health, purportedly signalling the Department's acceptance that hospital trusts would not necessarily be required to supply a full range of core services, and that even though there would continue to be a responsibility for the provision of a full range of core services locally, the precise definition of 'local' remained to be determined.[68]

With the passage of time, however, the issue of core services lost much of its emotive intensity. In order to avoid the charge of potentially important services failing to be defined as 'core' services in some districts, the Department of Health changed the nomenclature to 'designated' services, on the ground that 'core' services were misleadingly understood to be of special importance or priority.[21] 'Designated' services came to be defined simply as those which a DHA had deemed it necessary to be provided locally and where the only feasible provider was an NHS trust. In these limited circumstances the DHA could impose a contract upon a hospital trust for the provision of the designated services, with the Secretary of State having reserve powers of direction as a last resort. The issue was thereby placed into cold storage for the time being, doubtless available to be reheated in the event of the market showing signs of failing to provide easy local access to essential services.

Doubts about the capacity of the internal market to consolidate and extend the gains in social equality that the NHS had secured were a further thread in the fabric of concern about the regressive effects of *Working for Patients*. While the NHS had, in intent if not always in reality, provided an approximate equality of access to services of approximately equal standard for patients with approximately corresponding needs, the internal market might unstitch some of what had been achieved in the past and introduce new forms of inequality. Many examples were raised. Geographical inequalities would increase if patients in some parts of the UK were required to travel longer distances for care than those in other parts. They would also widen in unpredictable ways if the expansion of successful hospitals and the contraction or closure of unsuccessful ones was geographically patterned. Hospitals themselves would, as Lord Trafford pointed out in the House of Lords immediately following the publication of the White Paper, find their homogeneity of clinical standards eroded as the most talented doctors were attracted towards the most successful hospitals able to offer the highest rewards.[69] (That this prognostication was made by Lord Trafford was of interest not merely because he was a doctor but also because he was later appointed as Minister of State for Health with the specific task of steering the National Health Service and Community Care Bill through the House of Lords.) The random siting of the budget-holding general practices would allow some but not all patients a possible choice of the agency purchasing care on their behalf. Any success on the part of the budget-holding practices in negotiating contracts with hospitals embodying favourable terms and conditions of treatment would be to the disadvantage of patients registered with non budget-holding practices. The concentration of independent hospital facilities in the southern regions of Britain would offer more choice in those regions as the distinctions between the public and private sectors became increasingly blurred. In short, much of what had been achieved throughout the lifetime of the NHS in evening out the availability and quality of care would, it was feared, risk being lost in the commercial and competitive ethos of the market. The claim advanced by Mr Waldegrave[70] that the reforms would actually assist the health authorities in tackling inequalities in the service failed to carry much widespread conviction.

Linked to these concerns about equality were those of the possible conflicts that might arise between the imperatives of the market and the desirability of local participation and accountability. While the NHS could never claim to have been a truly participative service, the existing composition of the health authorities and the openness of their meetings, together with the rights and responsibilities accorded to the community health councils, had enabled a measure of local involvement in the provision and management of services and had ensured a kind of accountability to local communities. *Working for Patients* paid lip-service to the continuing engagement of local interests in the running of the NHS, but widespread concern was expressed that the proposed reforms would diminish even the muted elements of participation that currently existed because of the emphasis they gave to managerial rather than to public accountability.

Much of the concern centred upon the proposed changes to the membership of the DHAs (designed to transform them into the local agencies of the NHS Management Executive by enhancing their management strength at the expense of their representational functions), and upon the composition of the boards of directors of the NHS trusts. Gone from the DHAs would be the members appointed by the local authorities and those representing the trade unions and the medical and nursing constituencies in the districts. In their stead would be five executive and five non-executive members (the latter appointed solely for the relevance of their skills and experience), together with a non-executive chairman. The only medically qualified member would normally be the district director of public health. The boards of directors of the NHS trusts would be similarly constituted, their accountability lying directly with the Secretary of State. There was no requirement for the boards to meet in public or for their affairs to be open to public scrutiny. Indeed, the fear was expressed that the cloak of commercial secrecy would render some of the information and data about the operations of the NHS even less accessible to the public than hitherto.[71]

The diminishing emphasis given in *Working for Patients* to the involvement and participation of local communities in their health services merely served to emphasize the importance of the consultative machinery.[72] If people had little opportunity to influence the development of their local services, they ought at least to have access to fora in which their opinions could be expressed and heeded. The community health councils (CHCs) were seen to have an obvious role to play in this matter, as were also the myriad of patients' groups; but the signs were not propitious. A draft document reportedly leaked from the Department of Health in April 1990 revealed the government's intention to avoid any consultation with the CHCs over the creation of NHS trusts or the closure of hospitals, save where issues arose about the disposal of land or buildings.[73] The document reportedly characterized the existing consultation procedures as an 'obstacle to effective management' and noted the 'convenience' of changing the regulations to exempt all trust applicants from the statutory requirement to consult the CHCs. Regulations subsequently laid before Parliament announced that CHCs would have no formal role in monitoring the contracts set up for the provision of services, nor would they enjoy automatic visiting rights to non-NHS premises.[74] No mention was made of the budget-holding general practices. The treatment of the CHCs sat rather uncomfortably alongside the White Paper's rhetoric about the importance of consumer participation, and it naturally failed to please the councils and their supporters.[75] 'There will be no consumer scrutiny of purchasing decisions by GP budget-holders,' protested the Director of the Association of Community Health Councils, 'no mechanism to ensure that service standards and quality are built into the contracts between GPs and service providers, and no guarantee even that CHCs will be able to monitor the services purchased in this way.'

The final major area in which it was feared that *Working for Patients* might undermine the gains achieved by the NHS, that of the quality of trust between doctor and patient, depended for its effect (as did a number of the other issues discussed above) upon a rosy interpretation of how things had actually been in the NHS. A great strength of the NHS, so it was claimed, was the freedom of doctors to behave in ways that best met the needs of their patients, insulated from any direct responsibility for the financial consequences of their clinical decisions. *Working for Patients*, it was prophesied, would change all of that by making doctors more aware of, and accountable for, the cost of the resources they commanded. The prophecy was directed particularly towards the GPs, for whom the mandatory imposition of indicative drug budgets and the voluntary assumption of practice budgets would provide a fiscal corset of a kind they had not hitherto been obliged to wear. The effect on their relationships with their patients might be adverse. Increased awareness of the costs of the drugs they prescribed might place them under pressure to withhold prescriptions that might otherwise have been issued, and the cost to the practice budget of sending patients to hospital might likewise adversely affect their referral behaviour. If such outcomes were to occur, and if GPs were thought as a result to be compromising on the quality of their service in order to meet their budgetary targets, the trust between themselves and their patients would be eroded. Patients would lose confidence that they were receiving the best treatments for their needs as the suspicion deepened that doctors were basing their decisions as much upon financial as upon clinical criteria.

The fear was as much one of perception as of reality. Resources in the NHS have always fallen short of the level that could beneficially be used, and doctors have always in consequence been obliged to constrain their clinical freedoms within the resources available to them. The popular depiction of GPs as gatekeepers is a precise reflection of the control they exert over people's access to other parts of the NHS. There was nothing in *Working for Patients* that would alter this essential role: resources would continue to be tight, and doctors would continue, through their professional judgements and actions, to determine which patients gained access to which kinds of care. Even the introduction of indicative drug budgets was not the thoroughly innovative measure that many supposed, for GPs had always been open to corrective pressures if their prescribing costs were markedly out of line with those of their peers, and the pilot schemes introduced in 1988 to apprise GPs of the costs of their prescribing were, by early 1990, beginning to show signs of reducing the numbers of high-spending doctors.[76] It was possible to claim, however, that doctors had been sufficiently distanced from such influences to avoid the charge of being directly swayed by them in their daily work. Their covert role as rationers of care was not well understood by their patients, and most GPs would probably have denied the dominance of budgetary pressures over their care of individual patients. *Working for Patients*, by contrast, was designed in part to make the rationing process more explicit, more conscious and more visible by heightening the transparency to individual doctors (and hence, possibly, to their patients) of the financial implications of their work; and it was the effect of this upon the relationships between doctors and patients that caused concern.

Unsurprisingly, it was the Royal College of General Practitioners (RCGP) that took a leading role in the pursuit of this particular argument: in April 1989 the College Council rejected the White Paper on the grounds, *inter alia*, that 'if implemented as proposed, it will seriously damage patient care and the doctor–patient relationship'.[77] In the same month the Special Conference of Representatives of Local Medical Committees endorsed the RCGP's concern about the compromising effect that practice budgets would exert upon clinical practice,[65] and the Special Representative Meeting of the BMA in the following month did likewise.[78] Unsurprising also were the anecdotal stories appearing in the national press of patients with expensive drug requirements being refused admission to GPs' lists or even being requested to change to other practices.[79] If the introduction of budgets into general practice was to work for the benefit of patients, care would be needed in setting the budgets initially, and explicit guidelines would have to be drawn up about the division of responsibility for prescribing between the GPs and the hospital doctors.

7

IMPLEMENTATION

The two years and two months that elapsed between the publication of *Working for Patients* and the implementation of the Act of Parliament that gave expression to its ideals were witness to a complex and fluctuating series of manoeuvres, akin perhaps to a dance-floor upon which a mazurka, a progressive barn dance, an excuse-me and a game of musical chairs were all proceeding simultaneously, with nobody to conduct the orchestra. The British Medical Association and its fellow-travellers in protest pursued their imaginative campaigns of opposition to the White Paper in the manner and for the reasons described in the preceding chapters. Mr Clarke, the Secretary of State until his replacement by Mr Waldegrave in November 1990, defended the proposals in the White Paper with rumbustious vigour and created the political environment in which their implementation became possible. Parliament debated and eventually passed the necessary legislation to enable the changes to be made. Many component parts of the NHS were cajoled or enticed into reformulating themselves into the skeletal structures of the internal market. Public opinion, doubtless rendered punch-drunk by the onslaught of conflicting propaganda to which it was exposed, continued to entertain doubts about the wisdom of the whole thing and remained stubbornly convinced of the existence of a hidden agenda to privatize the NHS. And as the clock ticked away the weeks and months remaining to the next general election, the government undertook innumerable changes of mind and emphasis while usually denying that any such thing was happening. What emerged at the end of the process was a structural revision to the NHS that was very close indeed to the bare-bones specifications in *Working for Patients*, but an operational style that was far removed from the vision of the open and competitive market that had seemingly captivated its authors.

The influence of Mr Clarke and of his ministers and senior managers was crucial in the early stages of the process to ensure that the White Paper's implementation was not impeded by fruitless debate. The political risks of timing were severe: to introduce the internal market into the NHS would be complex and hazardous, liable (if the timing went wrong) to throw up embarrassing teething problems in the approach to the general election in 1991 or 1992.[1] Mr Clarke was, moreover, already under pressure to reach a swift conclusion in his negotiations with the general practitioners over their new contract.[2] Although few points of overlap existed between the White Paper and the GP contract (the most notable being the requirement for GPs to compete for patients by raising the proportion of their income derived from capitation payments), the disputations over the two documents proceeded in parallel, to the confusion of the general public at least. By March 1989, just as the BMA and the Department of Health were reaching a well-publicized stalemate over the GP contract,[3] the debate on the White Paper was getting nicely into its stride; and when *The Independent* carried the headline 'More doctors in threat to quit over reforms', it must have been far from clear to most of its readers which reforms were in question.[4] As the damaging confrontation over the GP contract dragged on through the spring and summer of 1989, seemingly jeopardizing the government's chances of securing public acceptance of the White Paper, the pressures increased on Mr Clarke both to reach a speedy conclusion on the contract and to show progress in implementing *Working for Patients*.[5] In the short term, the former proved the less tractable of the two, for although Mr Clarke had concluded a pact with the GPs' leaders by mid-May,[6] the deal was later rejected by the Conference of Local Medical Committees and by the GPs themselves, and the new contract had eventually to be imposed upon a resentful profession.[7]

If his public and sometimes bruising encounters with the GPs caused the Secretary of State to entertain second thoughts about the White Paper, it certainly did not show. Appearing often to be positively enjoying himself, Mr Clarke repeatedly and robustly defended the proposals to the House, to the Commons Social Services Committee and to the media, insisting in the process that the timetable laid out in *Working for Patients* (requiring the first hospital trusts, the first budget-holding general practices, the indicative drug budget scheme and the embryonic internal market to be up and running by 1991) would not be abandoned.[8] Two tactics were used openly to ensure adherence to the timetable: the outright refusal to contemplate pilot studies or demonstration projects as preludes to the nation-wide introduction of the market; and the minimization of consultation to avoid the risk of the local rejection of key changes.

The speed and dedication with which the government pursued its aims, together with its steadfast rejection of calls for experimentation, were a source initially of surprise and then of anger. It had been regarded almost as axiomatic, prior to the publication of the White Paper, that the internal market would have a limited introduction and be the subject of careful evaluation before its fiefdom was extended. The National Association of Health Authorities, in its evidence to the Prime Minister's review group, had advocated the gradual development of the internal market through a series of trials.[9] Academic commentators, including those who were broadly favourable to the principle of market competition in the NHS, argued likewise for the experimental testing of the viability of provider markets.[10] The East Anglian Regional Health Authority actually offered itself to the Department of Health in 1988 as a test-bed site.[11] Press speculation in the period leading up to the publication date took it almost for granted that alternative forms of market organization would be proposed in the White Paper for evaluation, and the BMA declared itself adamant that 'the government must not introduce changes without carrying out properly evaluated pilot studies'.[12] Even in the post-publication period, as ministers sought to make a virtue of the fact that the political impetus would not be compromised by the inevitable delays accompanying experimentation and trial, doctors and others continued to rehearse the case for pilot studies and demonstration projects. Among them was Professor Enthoven, who lent support to the cause of evaluation by declaring his enthusiasm for demonstration projects and describing the government's refusal to entertain them as a 'mistake'.[13]

Ministers responded by adapting their language while maintaining the brisk timetable of implementation. By mid-May 1989 Mr Clarke, though continuing to deny the need for 'formalised or academic monitoring or evaluation',[14] was assuring the House of Commons Social Services Committee of the intrinsically experimental nature of the whole thing from which lessons would be learnt and to which necessary changes would be made.[15] 'I don't recognise complaints that we're banging things into place just like that', he was reported as saying. 'We're actually evolving them steadily.' That was not, however, a view that was widely shared. As the year progressed, concern about the wisdom and realism of the government's timetable increased. The Department's Chief Medical Officer described the time allowed for consultation as 'very tight'.[16] An academic commentator dismissed the timespan allowed for the creation of the requisite information systems as 'clearly nonsense'.[17] The Society of Family Practitioner Committees expressed concern that the government had underestimated the mammoth commitment into which it was entering.[18] Professor Enthoven remarked upon the 'amazing speed' with which the internal market was to be introduced.[13] The Chartered Association of Certified Accountants spoke of the government's 'extremely ambitious timetable'.[19] The House of Commons Social Services Committee feared that, if the White Paper's timetable was adhered to, 'the stability of services and continuity of patient care may suffer during the years of transition to a new, untested system'.[20] Most wrathful of all, the editor of the *British Medical Journal* likened the government's tactics to those of 'steaming', a currently fashionable crime in which 'gangs run amok through a crowded train or carnival demanding money at knifepoint'.[21] The aim, the editor explained, 'is achieved through bewilderment and fear, much as in Clausewitz's description of total war'. Strong words indeed from an influential office!

Yet if the government's evident intent to press quickly ahead with the national implementation of *Working for Patients* without formal trial or experimentation caused widespread consternation and anger, only a little less ire was aroused by the second tactic enabling the brisk timetable to be maintained – the minimization of consultation. Many organizations, especially the medical ones, had plainly been affronted by their exclusion from the deliberations of the working group that prepared the White Paper, and they were in no mood for further marginalization. Yet although there was an obvious sense in which the government had no option but to heed the views of a wide spectrum of interests once the White Paper had been published, the feeling persisted and rankled in many quarters that the process was more akin to polite listening than to genuine consultation. Such feelings seemed to take as their case study the particular issue of local consultation over applications for NHS trust status.

The White Paper itself was silent on the obligation to consult about potential trusts, but the Working Paper on self-governing hospitals required successful applications for trust status to demonstrate that they 'carried the substantial commitment of those likely to be involved in the new management'. By way of amplification, the Secretary of State was reported as saying that 'we will want to be satisfied that there is a reasonable body of support among the hospital people and in the local community to make a go of it'.[22] Local managers concurred. By April 1989, however, reports were appearing of consultants voting against their local hospitals applying for trust status, and a survey by the BMA's Central Committee for Hospital Medical Services in June claimed that, of the 170 hospitals which had by then declared an interest in self-government, only one-third enjoyed the approval of their medical staffs.[23] The House of Commons Social Services Committee, in its major response to *Working for Patients* in August 1989, thought that local populations should be balloted before trust status was awarded,[24] and, as if to oblige, a random sample of residents in Doncaster were polled by MORI for their views on self-government for their local hospitals.[25] Sixty-eight per cent were opposed and only 13 per cent in favour. The pattern was emerging of seemingly widespread local opposition to the concept of NHS trusts while many hospitals were simultaneously preparing for just such a step.

The picture continued to develop as 1990 progressed. A survey published in February by the BMA's Central Consultants and Specialists Committee purported to show that the senior medical staff in 31 of 68 hospitals expecting to proceed with trust applications were undecided about the move, and in a further 19 they were opposed.[26] Of the 1,000 staff (out of 3,000) at Guy's and Lewisham hospitals participating in a ballot conducted by the Electoral Reform Society, 90 per cent were against self-government.[27] At St Bartholomew's Hospital, 81 of 160 consultants were opposed to the hospitals' intentions for trust status.[28] By June 1990, results were available from the ballots among consultants at 28 of the 79 hospitals regarded as likely to be among the first to apply for self-government: a majority was opposed to any such move in 19 of them and in favour in only 5.[29] Not only consultants, but also GPs and other health authority staff registered their opposition to self-governing status for their local hospitals. The seemingly growing divide between the sceptical and even hostile views of the doctors and the activities of many managers in preparing their applications for trust status threatened for a while to undermine the momentum towards the widespread dispersion of

NHS trusts. In response, the government appeared to modify its position on consultation: although a statutory period of consultation was to precede each application, Mr Clarke explained that its purpose was merely to assist him in deciding whether the application was in the best interests of the health service and its patients.[30] Later, in apparent contradiction to the assurances of the working paper on self-governing hospitals, he reportedly told a conference of the Institute of Health Services Management in June 1990 that the consultants in a hospital would not be able to veto its nomination as a trust.[29] Angry by this time at its failure to deflect the government from its chosen path (see Chapter 5), the medical profession could merely continue to fulminate at its impotence over the course of events, *The Lancet* denouncing the consultation period as 'phoney' and Mr Clarke's sanity as questionable.[31]

While the antagonists were weaving their patterns of protest upon the dance-floor, other and powerful movements were flowing around them to ensure that the major structures of *Working for Patients* would at least be in place (if not securely so) by the appointed date in April 1991. For all the apparent confusion and confrontation that pervaded the NHS in the wake of the White Paper, the impressive fact remains that the will of the politicians, the thraldom of the policy-makers and the collaboration of the managers held sufficiently firm throughout 1989 and 1990 to ensure that legislation was passed and acted upon that gave expression to almost all of the key proposals. It was, in many ways, a monumental achievement in the face of an unremittingly widespread opposition, effecting changes in structures, attitudes and working practices that might hitherto have been unimaginable within any timespan, least of all two years.

A key element was the early identification and mobilization of support where it existed. Potential hospitals and other trusts were identified by the regional health authorities and encouraged to declare themselves, and steps were taken to seek out possible first-wave budget-holding general practices.[32] Whatever early resistance there may have been to these twin innovations began gradually to thaw in the heat of the overtures made to them, yielding from an early date a small but steadily growing number of hospitals and general practices that came to be talked about as possible guinea-pigs in the new dispensation. Much of the process of persuasion was hidden from public gaze, but enough stories surfaced in the public arena to suggest that the time-honoured instruments of stick and carrot had probably not been locked irretrievably away in Departmental cupboards.

The sticks were, in the main, fiscal ones, several examples appearing in the public press of their determined use. A meeting of the General Medical Services Committee of the BMA in April 1989 heard accounts of hospitals being threatened with the loss of development funds if they failed to enthuse about self-government.[33] In May, consultants in the South West Thames region were said to be worried about the political and managerial pressures upon them to nominate their hospitals for trust status,[34] and reports emerged from Liverpool of the financial disadvantages that might attend the failure of hospitals to show an interest.[35] A consultant in Exeter wrote publicly of the exploitation of rivalries and of fear, greed and threats in the South Western region as 'the way in which the Department of Health is seeking to implement the NHS White Paper'.[36] The chairman of one RHA was reportedly accused by a consultant surgeon of threatening a group of doctors over the future of their hospital if they did not support an expression of interest in self-government.[37] Further whistles were blown in public by medical members of health authorities, in one case even accusing a district general manager of registering his district's formal expression of interest in self-government before the matter had actually been decided by the authority.[38] Such stories may or may not have been true in their entirety, but the very fact of their publication (some of them in the form of letters penned by the complainants themselves) gave a measure of the public estrangement that had grown up between governors and governed.

All was not negative, however: carrots were also spotted by the *cognoscenti*, though whether they existed in reality or only in the imagination was sometimes unclear. Part of the argument was that, since the eventual implementation of the White Paper was realized from an early date to be inevitable, many health authorities and hospitals felt themselves better able to protect their interests from the inside than the outside. Likewise, many GPs who were unsympathetic in principle to holding their own budgets quickly came to realize that, however bad budget-holding might prove to be, it was hardly likely to be worse than an enforced reliance upon the contracts placed for them by their district health authorities. Just as important, however, were the positive rewards that were believed to be available to those who took an early plunge. As the Nuffield Professor of Medicine at Oxford put the matter quite early in the debate, 'because of the considerable political advantages for the government if a large number of hospitals are seen to be moving to self-government by 1991, an early expression of interest may lead to preferential treatment in the interim'.[39] Stories began to emerge of hospitals becoming inquisitive about self-government as a way of avoiding closure, of gaining revenue, of acquiring new buildings, or of expunging debts. Whether any such inducements had indeed been proffered is not a matter for empirical verification, but complaints were certainly raised later about the first wave of hospital trusts having been misled about the favoured access they would enjoy to funds for capital developments.[40]

Not only potential trusts but also prospective budget-holding practices were thought likely to be offered incentives. As *The Guardian* put the point in an editorial, 'the first GPs who take up practice budgets will receive obvious benefits'.[41] The nature of the benefits became apparent in a Departmental document issued as a prospectus to potential budget-holding practices in December 1989.[42] Practices would receive a non-refundable allowance of £16,000 per practice to cover preparatory costs, an annual management allowance of £32,000, and the reimbursement of a higher proportion of computer maintenance costs than would be available to non budget-holding practices. Later, further incentives were offered to enable practices to install the computer systems required to manage their budgets.[43]

Along with the mobilization of the interest of prospective trust hospitals and budget-holding practices went the steady development of district structures, enabling the market to operate (in however shadowy a way) by the appointed day. The size and complexity of the tasks to be completed at district level, daunting under any circumstances, were magnified by the requirement to accomplish them within an astonishingly tight timetable while continuing to operate a normal service.[44] That the market was able to function in even a rudimentary fashion by April 1991 was a remarkable tribute to the quantity and quality of effort expended by staff at many different levels in the districts and boards. Purchasing teams had to be assembled to assess the local patterns of need for health care, to determine priorities, to develop indicators of the quantity and quality of the services they sought to purchase, and to begin the task of monitoring the impact of services on the health of their populations. Hospitals and other provider units had to have their management structures revised and strengthened, their lines of accountability clarified, and their financial and accounting systems overhauled to fit them for their new lives either as self-governing trusts or as directly managed units. Existing alliances within districts had to be reviewed and new ones created to enable the necessary interchanges and negotiations to occur between district managers, GPs, family health services authorities and local authorities. Better information than currently existed had to be assembled about local patterns of service use, especially hospital referrals, to enable contracts to be placed that would be acceptable to the GPs in the district. Prospective NHS trusts had to be identified and their contributions towards the district's purchasing requirements resolved. Financial and accounting strategies had to be reviewed and developed to cope with the revisions to the formula for the allocation of revenue resources and to create the structures for billing and handling the costs of the treatment of non-resident patients. Resource management had to be implemented in many hospitals. Purchasing requirements had to be specified in contractual terms and negotiated with the array of prospective providers. Control systems had to be established to ensure that contractual payments were made, quality criteria adhered to, and monitoring systems instituted. Methods had to be devised for recording, and paying for, the treatments given to patients referred to hospitals with which no prior contract existed. The old DHAs had to be decommissioned and the new ones appointed. And always the antagonists had to be confronted and the doubters reassured.

The detailed history of how the NHS underwent such a profound metamorphosis in the space of only 26 months will, in due course, be a work of its own. Though much of it proceeded behind the scenes, removed from public gaze and even from public understanding, intelligible controversies did appear from time to time. One was the problem of senior district managers caught between their dual responsibilities for both purchasing and providing (see Chapter 6); another was the charge of political bias in the appointment of members to the new health authorities;[45] and a third was the possibility (initially dismissed but later accepted by Mr Clarke) of entire districts opting for self-governing trust status, robbing the DHAs of all their functions as providers and managers. Of particular concern with the passage of time were the newly emerging patterns of inter-district and inter-agency networks that were thrown up from the loosening of former strictures and the dawning of new possibilities for self-determination. Although the White Paper made passing reference to possible future mergers among districts to enhance their purchasing power and scope, *Working for Patients* had no direct concern with structural change of this sort, nor was it foreseen in the early months of the debate. Yet along with the experience of creating the new district structures there came a growing realization of the virtual inevitability of the transformation of the 192 health districts in England and Wales (and their counterparts elsewhere in the UK) into a smaller number of large conglomerates.

One factor giving impetus to the trend was simply the shortage of skilled staff: not only were experienced managers and specialists in public health in short supply in several localities, but many of them also began to gravitate towards the provider side of the market, threatening to leave the purchasing authorities bereft of talent.[46] Mergers came to be seen as a necessary device for conserving and concentrating experienced staff. Moreover, the relatively large number of districts, combined with the relatively small size of their populations, might, if acting as single purchasers, create a fragmented and unnecessarily competitive network of purchasing agencies – the more so if they came to be competing with large numbers of budget-holding general practices. Many smaller purchasers would, according to one seasoned observer, be little short of disastrous, weakening their leverage in the market and increasing their subservience to the large providers.[47]

The force of this prediction was revealed in dramatic fashion by the experiences of the Rubber Windmill, the code-name of a management game played out in East Anglia in the spring of 1990, aimed at simulating the first three years of the internal market in the NHS (April 1990 to March 1993).[48] The 40 participants, including many with practical experience of contracting at departmental, regional and district levels, played out a variety of key professional roles in the contracting process in two health districts which, though fictitious, mimicked real ones in the region. Three hours of the game represented one year of the market. The Rubber Windmill was said later to have been influential in moderating a number of features of the actual implementation of the market in the NHS, not least because of the political turbulence caused by the widespread publicity given to its central conclusion – that the market collapsed as unworkable in the third year of the simulation. Prominent among the reasons for the collapse were the influential but idiosyncratic purchasing policies being pursued by the budget-holding general practices and (rather surprisingly) the local authorities, forcing the DHAs into a kind of crisis management as the financial pressures accumulated in the second and third years. 'To tackle this problem', the Rubber Windmill concluded, 'it becomes essential to forge some consistent and coherent strategic framework for purchasing between local authorities, health authorities and general practitioners.'[48] To this list was later added the family health services authorities (FHSAs) as they began to evolve into primary care authorities with a potential purchasing role of their own.

Developments on the ground matched (and in some cases anticipated) the emerging consensus on the inevitability of commissioning clusters composed of two or more DHAs and possibly also of FHSAs. In August 1989 the first report appeared of a plan to create a commissioning cluster in south-east London,[49] and by the end of the following year exploratory talks on joint purchasing agencies were reportedly taking place in several regions.[50] Amid forecasts of a future NHS in England comprising perhaps 90 large purchasing groups each of the size of the old area health authorities, the NHS Management Executive (ME) began explicitly to encourage the regional general managers to integrate the work of their DHAs and FHSAs.[51] The pattern, though clearly evolving, was not unanimously approved, however. Fears were expressed about the remoteness of the clusters from their local communities, about their lack of public accountability, and about the untested assumptions of the benefits of scale they would generate. To these was added a distinctly economic note: the larger and the fewer the commissioning clusters, the greater would be the distortions caused to the market through the presence of powerful oligopsonies able to impose their interests on the smaller providers who would be dependent upon their custom.[52] Once again the tensions emerged between the realities of managing the market, on the one hand, and the freedom of the market to yield its beneficial outcomes, on the other.

In parallel with the district transformations, the management structure within the Department of Health was also evolving into the new forms proposed in *Working for Patients*. In May 1989 the membership was revealed of the NHS Policy Board, chaired and appointed by the Secretary of State and charged with determining 'the strategy, objectives and finances of the service in the light of government policy'. Among the members appointed to the Board with no previous specialist experience of the NHS were a number of prominent industrialists, three of whom had earlier been involved in the restructuring of public sector industries preparatory to their transfer to the private sector. Understandably, they were represented (though in truth probably misrepresented) as harbingers of what might befall the NHS.[53] In May also the membership of the

ME was appointed. Chaired by the Chief Executive, Mr Nichol, the ME was designed as the executive powerhouse of the service, translating the aspirations of the Policy Board into purposeful action by the regions, districts and boards. Its position at the pinnacle of the hierarchy of command and obedience created in the wake of the White Paper endowed it, almost inevitably, with a political aura that it ought not to have had, being technically part of the Civil Service. Excluded from membership were the Department's Chief Medical Officer, Chief Nursing Officer and Director of Health Authority Finance; included were experienced NHS managers (including the Chief Executive) and a small number of specialists from backgrounds far removed from the NHS.

The result, as the *British Medical Journal* observed in a commentary upon the appointments, was the transfer of control over the service away from career Civil Servants towards 'streetwise NHS managers' – a change that might, with luck, achieve the long-cherished goal of a central focus for the management of the NHS, free from the day-to-day political influence of ministers.[54] That this was not to be became apparent early in 1991 with the announcement of further changes to the ME in the wake of a report from the Executive's Director of Operations and Planning depicting the ME as 'an organisation very well designed to provide advice to ministers – but not designed to manage the health service'.[55] The changes, planned to coincide with the relocation of the ME from London to Leeds in 1992, were aimed in part at freeing the ME from the control of ministers, allowing it to 'manage the NHS with clear credibility and leadership' – an aim that was of great significance in establishing and maintaining the momentum of change initiated by the White Paper. Yet ambiguity remained about the relationship between the Management Executive and the Department's traditional staff of Civil Servants, and more pointedly between the Chief Executive and the Department's Permanent Secretary – an ambiguity that was heightened rather than alleviated by the announcement of the shift to Yorkshire.[56] Echoing the fragmentation of management control at the local level was a cognate dispersion of power at the centre. The notion of a *national* health service was steadily being lost.

The fruits of the government's punishing timetable for the implementation of *Working for Patients* ripened one by one as the months ticked by. In February 1989 the first eight working papers were published and names were beginning to emerge of hospitals likely to be among the front runners for trust status. By May, 140 expressions of interest in trust status had been registered, rising in the next month to 178. In July the Department of Health issued a further working paper on capital charging and a guide to self-governing hospitals. By November, when the National Health Service and Community Care Bill was published, 79 hospitals and units were actively preparing their trust applications. At the end of 1989, no fewer than 34 project groups, sponsored by the Department, were at work on many facets of implementation. In January 1990 the prospectus on general practice budget-holding was issued to woo prospective practices, and expressions of interest in budget-holding were beginning to emerge. The Department's strategy for information technology in the new NHS was unveiled at the end of January, shortly before the Bill went to the committee stage. In March 1990, as 880 general practices were lodging an interest in holding their own budgets and possible candidates for trust status in the second wave were beginning to identify themselves, the Bill was guillotined through the committee stage and the Secretary of State announced that all services would be delivered through contracts by 1991. In May the Department's guide to the development of districts was published and details of the new consultants' contract unveiled. The Bill received Royal Assent in June, and leaflets were sent to the general public explaining the benefits it would bring. In September the new health authorities came into being. In October, as the consultation period ended for the first wave of trust applications, expressions of interest were being registered by prospective second-wave trusts. The first 57 trusts were announced shortly before Christmas, and following the festive break the RHAs began to negotiate practice budgets with 312 practices (of which all but six were confirmed in March as the first wave of budget-holding practices). By the time the Act came into force, on 1 April 1991, the skeletal structures of the internal market were visibly in place, and were almost exactly those that had been sketched out over two years earlier in *Working for Patients*.

Yet behind the outward show of a smooth and purposeful movement towards the ordained goal lay a great deal of chaos, confusion and uncertainty. It was as though the government had unleashed a hurricane of reforming energy whose force and direction could be controlled only in the broadest way. At all levels of the service – regional, district and unit – new freedoms appeared and new possibilities were created for those who wished to break the moulds of inherited structures and practices, to forge new frameworks and alliances, to assume fresh responsibilities and to create novel options and opportunities. It was inevitable in such an energetic, entrepreneurial and innovative environment that mistakes should be made, judgements should be clouded, corners should be cut, morale should be impaired, and deviations should occur from the intended track. If an omelette cannot be made without breaking the proverbial eggs, then forty years of established practices and attitudes within the nation's largest organization certainly could not be altered without an enormous amount of turbulence, uncertainty, chaos, anger and fear. To depict the implementation of *Working for Patients* as a carefully planned or controlled progression would be wholly inaccurate.

A flavour of the complexity, confusion and protest whipped up by the White Paper has been conveyed in this and preceding chapters. To this must be added the government's repeated changes of mind and emphasis, less on matters to do with the structure of the market (though many of these occurred) than with its ways of working. For behind the outwardly confident assertions of the government and its supporters about the beneficial effects of market competition in enhancing efficiency and generating greater value for money, steps were progressively being taken to ensure that the new internal market of the NHS would actually generate very little competition, and almost none at all in its early days.

Of the government's original intention to create a genuinely competitive market there can be little doubt: *Working for Patients* was the ambitious product of a political environment that preferred private to public domains, markets to bureaucracies, competition to patronage, and individual choice to social equality. The language of ministers and of Departmental documents in the months immediately following the White Paper's publication was unmistakably that of commercial discourse, and for as long as Mrs Thatcher remained in Downing Street there seemed to be little doubt about the long-term direction in which the NHS was intended to head. Yet the chorus of protest against the ideological thrust of the Paper, though outwardly effecting little apparent influence over the legislative course of events, was finally not bereft of all political leverage, for as fortunes swayed in the propaganda battle for the hearts and minds of the people, so the language of the government's spokesmen moderated and their explicit commitment to the values of the market began to recede. The shifting use of language was perhaps the clearest public signal of the attitudinal transformations that were taking place.[57] What were 'buyers' in the White Paper became, with the passage of time, purchasers and then commissioners. 'Sellers' became providers. 'General practice budgets' became general practice funds. 'Indicative drug budgets' became indicative amounts. 'Contracts' became service agreements. 'Self-governing hospitals' became trusts. 'Marketing' became needs assessment. 'Pilot studies' became demonstration sites and then locality projects. Most telling of all, the initial introduction of the market, destined originally to bring about the most fundamental changes ever engineered in the NHS, came to be depicted as a time of 'steady state', implying a smoothly progressive continuity with the past rather than a sharp divergence from it.

The retreat from the aggressive language of the early months, begun while Mr Clarke was still in office, lost all pretence of concealment when he was replaced as Secretary of State by Mr Waldegrave early in November 1990. Speaking with disarming candour at the Royal College of Surgeons in December, Mr Waldegrave reportedly charged the government with having been carried away in its application of business language to the NHS, causing alarm to 'quite a lot of people who think that we do not know the difference between a hospital and a supermarket'.[58] While insisting upon the need to sharpen the management of the service, Mr Waldegrave reportedly conceded that 'we have overdone the language of commerce. Without remitting for one moment the pressure to get a better management system, let us watch our language a bit'. Nor was it only the language that moderated: lacking Mr Clarke's cheerfully pugnacious approach to his adversaries, Mr Waldegrave adopted a studiedly more conciliatory approach towards the doctors, acceding to the BMA's request for confidential talks with himself and the Prime Minister about the progress of the reforms and eliciting in return the Association's renunciation of its high-profile campaign of confrontation with the government.[59]

Nor was the sea-change merely one of style: as the appointed day approached, the management of the market became increasingly heavy, ensuring that, for a while at least, it would produce no alarming or embarrassing outcomes that could give political capital to the government's opponents. Freedoms that had earlier been proclaimed as vital to the effective functioning of the market failed to materialize in ways expected, and the much vaunted vision of a service offering greater choice was rapidly becoming a mirage. Early in 1991 *The Economist* proclaimed:

> The Department of Health is on the defensive, plagued by stories of hard-done-by patients and terrified by words like 'market' and 'competition' . . . In order to avoid an election-losing shake-up the new market will be strictly controlled from the centre . . . The government is terrified that the idea at the heart of the reforms – making money follow the patient – might increase efficiency but lose votes.[60]

Many areas of the market were affected (and in some cases disaffected) by the changing instructions coming down from on high. The freedom promised by the White Paper to the NHS trusts of employing staff on their own locally negotiated terms and conditions began to erode with the exclusion of junior hospital doctors (who would remain employed on national terms), continued with a Departmental warning to the trusts to avoid excessive salary payments to their chief executives, and escalated in June 1991 with a reported claim by the government of its willingness to accept national terms and conditions for *all* doctors employed in trust hospitals in exchange for the BMA's cessation of its opposition to the trusts.[61] Not only were the trusts' freedoms of employment the subject of nibbling erosion, but so also were their powers of raising capital. The veiled promise of greater access to funds for capital development had seemingly been an important incentive in the quest for trust status, and many hospitals had offered themselves in the first wave in the expectation of preferential treatment.[62] In the event, the borrowing limits placed upon the first wave of trusts were only a little more generous than those allowed to other hospitals, and their originating debt was split between public dividend capital and interest-bearing debt in a much less advantageous way than had been expected.[63] Predictably, many trust managers complained that they had been misled by the Department of Health about their borrowing and repayment capacities;[40] though since any such borrowing would effectively constitute an increase in the public sector borrowing requirement, the trusts were never likely to enjoy unlimited access to capital funds.

General practitioners were also the recipients of conflicting messages as the political repercussions of the market began to emerge. Assurances that had earlier been given to non fund-holding GPs about their continued freedom to refer their patients to hospitals of their choice were steadily withdrawn as the exercise of such freedoms began to conflict with the contractual obligations entered into by their DHAs. By the spring of 1991 reports were appearing of the imposition on GPs of restricted referral options,[64] and by the summer the possibility was arising of some DHAs running out of money to pay for the referrals that GPs were making outwith the existing contracts.[65] A tension was building up between the logic of the market and the clinical freedom of the doctors that seemed likely further to test the nerve and commitment of the government, especially as the 'steady state' gave way to a more dynamic disposition and contracts came increasingly to be placed with other than the traditional providers.

The fund-holding general practices enjoyed a degree of immunity from this particular tension, but they, too, were caught up in the policy changes that characterized the early days of the market. Virtuous capital had been made in the White Paper of their freedom to determine their own priorities for their patients and to secure the best deals on their behalf; but the bloom began to fade as evidence emerged of the inequalities resulting from the preferential services offered to patients of fund-holding practices and of the capacity of these practices to frustrate the attainment of local health targets by their unilateral purchases.[66] Early in 1991 the Department of Health requested the first wave of fund-holding practices not to depart from their historical referral patterns in placing their first contracts, and by the summer agreement had been reached between the Department and the BMA on guidelines to prohibit hospitals from lengthening the waiting times for some patients in order to offer speedier treatment to those referred from fund-holding practices.[67] A joint committee of the Department and the BMA's General Medical Services Committee was set up to study the impact of the fund-holding scheme on the treatment of all patients, wherever registered.

None of these changes of emphasis and practice amounted to a repudiation of the market, though they did represent a measure of retreat from the White Paper's enthusiastic espousal of market principles. It was becoming clear that the market would, initially at least, be managed and controlled in ways deemed likely to reduce the risks of unpalatable outcomes at a time of heightened political sensitivity towards the NHS. Perhaps the most explicit distancing from the White Paper's principles, however, was to be seen in the government's handling of hospital care in London – long regarded as the ultimate touchstone of the market's capacity to bring order and efficiency to a complex, expensive and over-resourced network of services.

The problems of London's hospitals sprang largely from the

existence in the capital of a large number of teaching and other hospitals offering a high capacity of beds and an expensive menu of services to a resident population that had been declining for many decades, but upon which the demand for care was boosted by the large numbers of daily commuters into the metropolis and by the waves of patients referred from other districts throughout the land. The problem had been concealed until 1974 by the teaching hospitals' insulation from the general system of hospital funding and by their access to trust funds and endowments, and since 1974 (though less successfully) by the adjustments made to the RAWP targets for the London districts to compensate them for their treatment of non-resident patients. The internal market of *Working for Patients*, however, threatened to blow the system apart: by funding the DHAs according to resident populations rather than patients treated, and by releasing the authorities to place their contracts with providers other than their local hospitals if that is what they wished to do, the efficiency of the teaching hospitals would be starkly exposed, and those that were unable to compete would suffer decline or even closure. London, with its large number of marginal Parliamentary constituencies, thus became a critical test of the government's faith in the market; for to hold faith might be to run the severe political risk of the contraction or even the demise of some of the best-known and most prestigious hospitals in the land.

The first sign of a possibly wavering faith came in December 1990, when the government decided to postpone the full implementation of the population-based formula for the allocation of revenue resources until 1992–3, when the next general election would be safely out of the way.[68] A safety net was announced for the interim period to protect localities that would have suffered under the impact of the unmoderated formula. London hospitals benefited. The forecasts of financial difficulties that the London hospitals might experience when required to compete in the market began to materialize in the spring of 1991 when the Guy's and Lewisham hospitals, which had received trust status in April, announced an inherited deficit of £6.8 million which the trust was planning to meet through the rationalization of services and the shedding of jobs.[69] The initial response of the government was faithful, arguing that that was what the market was designed to do, and that any intervention to limit the political damage would be an unwarranted intrusion.[70] Yet the government's second thoughts, influenced no doubt by the prospect of a general election within a year at most, were rather more apostatical: in October 1991 it announced that further applications for trust status from London hospitals would be deferred until a new commission of inquiry had reported upon the problems of hospital care in the capital.[71] The market was apparently not, after all, to be allowed to settle a problem that had defied bureaucratic attempts at solution for almost a century.

8

REFLECTIONS

The middle of a fast flowing river is not an ideal vantage point from which to judge the end towards which the waters are hurtling, least of all when a notice on the bank warns of a dangerous general election round the bend. Yet that was the position from which this concluding chapter was written, with at most seven months remaining until a general election, the outcome of which could determine the character of the NHS for many years. That such a possibility existed at all was a measure of the politicization the service had undergone: not only had the policies of the major political parties increasingly diverged, thrusting the NHS into the limelight of policy debate and party-political altercation, but also the policy-making machinery *within* the service had become ever more subject to governmental control to ensure the local implementation of central initiatives and to minimize the occurrence of politically embarrassing events. With the exception of a brief respite in 1990–1 caused by the dramatic changes in Downing Street and the momentous events in Kuwait, the NHS had rarely been out of the spotlight of media attention since the publication of *Working for Patients*, becoming the focus of increasingly acrimonious disputation as the general election loomed ever closer.

These uncertainties in the political landscape were not the only hazards in attempting a mid-stream assessment of the significance of *Working for Patients*. It had been all but impossible for ordinary members of the public to know exactly how the NHS had been changing since 1989. The tips of icebergs could be spotted, but not the masses below the water-line. Numerous local changes and developments had probably gone unreported; national structures had given way to a multiplicity of local variations as new groupings and alliances had emerged in different patterns in different places;

and a new air of secrecy and misprision had grown up. Reliance had inevitably to be placed upon journalistic sources of information that were themselves liable to partiality, sifting and presenting their information in ways most likely to advance the interests of their readers. The *British Medical Journal*, from which much of the material in the preceding chapters had been culled, had an obvious duty to represent and promote the interests of the medical profession; and the *Health Service Journal*, when charged with its persistently biased reporting of anything to do with the White Paper, retorted in an editorial that 'it is not the role of an independent press to smooth the way for government policy'.[1] Separating rhetoric from reality, froth from substance, was a further hazard. Fundamentally differing accounts had been offered in the media of the costs and benefits of the reforms as the combatants in the propaganda battle had fought for the allegiance of the people. Some said that *Working for Patients* had wrought substantial gains even in a matter of months, others that it had been an unmitigated disaster for the NHS, and still others that it had actually had very little effect one way or the other. The truth, if it could ever have been known, was bound to be incapable of containment within simple slogans, yet how could the 'truth' even be conceptualized, much less accessed?

The longer-term significance of *Working for Patients* can be seen in different lights by imagining alternative possible judgements that might be made about it in, say, five to ten years' time. In one light it might appear as a historical aberration – the product of a time-locked ideology that was already on the wane even as the Act came into force. Looking back from this perspective the White Paper may be seen as a late but genuine flowering of what had come to be called Thatcherism – the extension to the very heart of the welfare state of the principles of commercialization, competition and consumerism that provided the ideological glue to Mrs Thatcher's programmes of reform. As long as she remained in Downing Street, the NHS travelled remorselessly down the commercial path illuminated by the White Paper, and the longer the journey lasted, the greater the chances of irreversible shifts of attitudes and structures occurring. With Mrs Thatcher's replacement as Prime Minister by John Major, however, the style and content of government action began to change: the language of the competitive market gave way to that of public service, charters became more newsworthy than contracts, and what were seen by many as the wilder excesses of ideological fervour were tempered by the realities of electoral opinion. While the obituaries of Thatcherism could not be read with indecent haste, the word was quietly put around that the death had indeed occurred; and although the Thatcher years had been exhilarating for those who had commanded them, few had really expected them to last for ever.

The NHS, from this future perspective, might be seen as the unfortunate victim of a mugging that ought never to have occurred. Saddled at great cost with a market apparatus that nobody really wanted and that now would never be allowed to function in accordance with the manufacturer's specifications, it faces a rather bleak future. Heavily managed from the centre to ensure that localized sparks of interest in a competitive market are not permitted to ignite a bushfire of enthusiasm, the service will have to struggle on with trust hospitals that are supposed to behave as though they were independent businesses but in fact are not allowed to, with fund-holding general practices that are not able to decide for themselves how best to use their resources for their patients' benefit, and district health authorities that are partly purchasers and partly providers but not wholly either.

In another future light, *Working for Patients* might be seen as a seminal document that, far from being a mugger's weapon, is now widely recognized as the incisive blade that cut the Gordian knots entangling the NHS since 1948. Of course it was a shade extravagant in its language and its claims, but that was a necessary price to pay for the initiation of change in an organization noted more for inertia than for impetus. Of course it encountered all manner of teething problems in its early days, but that was an inevitable consequence of systemic change in a huge bureaucracy. Yet the principles of the White Paper were well founded; they eventually fired the enthusiasm of staff of all disciplines and all grades in the NHS who saw in them a genuine means towards a better service; and they raised a head of steam for reform that the political process could not have constrained for long even if it had tried to do so. The internal market is, naturally, managed in ways that minimize the risk of unwanted outcomes, but not so heavily as to snuff out all possibility of the achievement of genuine gains in efficiency through the benign effects of competition. *Working for Patients* is not, from this future perspective, seen as an exercise in the blind application of ideology; rather, it is viewed as the replacement of one set of principles for managing a public service industry with another better attuned to the spirit and technologies of the time. Once the political froth had cleared and the expected improvements began to show, the virtues of the market were recognized and appreciated; and people now marvel that it could ever have been the cause of such antagonism.

The future for the NHS in this light is rosy but possibly unpredictable. If the market is allowed to do its work, and if it continues to produce the goods that its supporters have promised, then the future will indeed be better than the past. Resources will be put to more efficient use; the quality of the caring process will rise; choice will be extended; and the health of the people will improve. Yet markets develop their own momentum, and the internal market in the NHS, if permitted to flourish, may evolve in ways that are unforeseen and possibly unwanted. It is here that the real risks of privatization may lie – not as the purposeful act of a government bent on the wholesale transfer of publicly owned resources to the private sector, but as the irresistible outcome of pressure from those whose behaviour is increasingly entrepreneurial and who demand a commensurately commercial environment in which to work.

In yet another future light, *Working for Patients* might be valued less for what it contained than for what it initiated. The more extreme commercial attitudes of the White Paper were never likely to last for long, and the market structures that it championed were so ill suited to the ethos of the NHS that their widespread acceptance was always in doubt. What it did achieve, however, was the destabilization of existing structures and processes from which a new form of service planning and management was enabled to emerge. The positive elements in the White Paper (such as the development of audit and information technology and the refinement of costing systems and outcome measurements) were beneficially integrated into the existing machinery; the divorce between the commissioning and the providing of services was carried through in ways that transformed health assurance from a fashionable slogan into a substantive process; the amalgamations between the district health authorities and the family health services authorities and their new relationships with the regional health authorities enabled an integrated approach to planning that had hitherto been unattainable; and the deflection of central management responsibility for the NHS away from the Department's Civil Servants towards the free-standing Management Executive released the service from the tyranny of political control over its day-to-day workings. That the trust hospitals and the fund-holding general practices eventually came to nought was neither here nor there: they were logical but ultimately unacceptable elements of an audacious plan that had to be shocking to unravel much of the existing fabric of the NHS and recreate it in new forms.

The future of the NHS from this perspective, once the dust has finally settled over the painful process of transition, looks good. The essential principles and frameworks of the service have been preserved and the divisive prospect of a commercial market averted, but much has been learnt in the process of change, and fresh attitudes and practices have been allowed to flourish. A step has also been taken down the ladder of politicization, releasing the NHS from the worst excesses of inter-party squabbling that were evident in the early 1990s. Whether there will be measurable gains in the efficiency of the component services and in the quality of the care they deliver (and, if so, whether they will be greater than a competitive market could have produced) will doubtless continue to be a matter of heated debate.

In yet another future light, *Working for Patients* might be largely forgotten by all except the academics and historians, going the way of other similarly titled documents (such as *Patients First*[2]) whose contents can no longer be recalled and whose influence on the NHS is obscure. The internal market has collapsed, largely because of the unsustainably high transaction costs, but nothing of substantial novelty has been put in its place. The NHS has gradually been allowed to drift back to its pre-1989 position, the White Paper being blamed for most of its manifestations of continuing malaise. The future is bleak.

Whatever may be the judgement of future generations on *Working for Patients*, a provisional balance sheet of its credits and debits to date can be drawn up. The credits appear to be substantial. First, it has released many constraints against change, and has begun to replace inertia with impetus. While few if any of the primary objectives of the White Paper were new, and most could have been achieved without resort to the structural changes mandated in the 1990 Act, the wheels of change in the NHS have often turned rather slowly. Now their rotation is noticeably brisk. Whether the outcome will be judged in time to be, on balance, beneficial or otherwise remains to be seen; but that transformations are occurring at an unprecedented rate is indubitable.

Second, the changing ethos in the NHS is encouraging and allowing initiative and innovation. Managers are enjoying a field day as they review and revise their existing ways of doing things, create new alignments and alliances, and explore possibilities that have hitherto been barred from consideration by institutional obstacles. Tackling the oversupply of hospital beds in London is one example of this loosening of constraints. While the government's apparent refusal to accept the outworkings of the market may be seen as a loss of political nerve, the new atmosphere has forced the institution of a long-overdue review of the capital's needs and resources. More generally, the new alliances that have had to be forged at district level may eventually succeed in bringing a greater integration to the NHS than any of the great post-war reorganizations had managed to achieve. That DHAs are now having to consult the GPs practising within their boundaries, and are finding it necessary to create joint commissioning arrangements with the FHSAs, is likely to be of lasting benefit; yet it may not have happened within such a short space of time but for the destabilization and subsequent realignments caused by the White Paper.

Third, a renewed impetus has been given to the development of the information systems that ought to be underpinning a modern health care system, whether or not it is organized along commercial lines. Costing systems are being developed with a new urgency. Issues about the quality of care are being considered in a more explicit way than hitherto. Methods of assessing a population's needs for health care and of judging the impact of services upon health status are being developed with new intent. Systems for auditing the quality of care, both in hospitals and in primary care, are being created (if not yet fully exploited) on a scale that has not hitherto been attained. The quest for relevant and timely information, for both clinical and management purposes, has acquired a new urgency and has attracted a new level of resource investment.

Fourth, the distinction between the commissioning and the providing of care, however it may eventually be managed, has succeeded in principle in transferring power away from those with vested interests in the maintenance of clinically interesting domains towards those with a more global outlook. It should become less easy for clinicians in the prestigious and powerful specialties to appropriate for themselves an unreasonable share of a district's resources, and *pari passu*, it could enable more funding to be directed towards service areas (such as prevention and priority care) that have previously suffered in the scramble for resources by their lack of political leverage. Whether the commissioners will succeed in freeing themselves from the dominance of the prestigious providers and develop a more balanced portfolio of contracts remains to be seen; but the commissioning agencies have at least been given the opportunity and the authority to reorientate their thinking away from the provision of services towards the assurance of health, and to determine their service priorities in the light of global objectives for the health of their people.

Fifth, issues about choices and priorities have become more open and explicit. The need for the rationing of resources and care has not diminished, for the NHS will remain a service in which a cash-limited volume of resource is required to be allocated among a plethora of competing needs, not all of which can be met at an acceptable standard of care. Governments will still be required to share a finite cake among the regions and the regions among the districts; the districts and the fund-holding general practices will still be required to select their priorities from among the hospital and community health services; and the clinicians will still be required to ration the allocation of their time and attention among the patients requiring them. Yet these stages of the rationing process may, in some respects, become more visible and, therefore, more open to contestation. In particular, if the public is allowed access to the contracts placed by the DHAs and the fund-holding general practices, people's awareness of local priorities should be raised, providing ammunition to those who may wish to challenge them. At a national level, the availability of better information about the costs and outcomes of the service may, as ministers have always conceded, strengthen the arguments of those who believe the NHS to be badly underfunded.

So much, in brief, for the credits. The provisional debits are no less impressive. The deeply contested nature of the White Paper's proposals and the speed at which they have been imposed upon a reluctant service may have sown the seeds of a confusion and hostility that will yield a harvest of bitterness for years to come. The alienation of staff from their managers, the mistrust of politicians by the electorate, and the fears of patients about the primacy of financial considerations in the choice of their treatments may be causing extensive damage to the fabric of goodwill in which the NHS has traditionally been wrapped, and that may take years to restore. Moreover, the obviously growing politicization of the service, with the threat of major policy reversals at every future change of government, bodes ill for the continuity and development of the NHS along channels directed towards the good of the people. In the short term, at least, a rational debate about the complicated problems facing the NHS and the complexity of the means by which they may be addressed has given way to dogmatic assertions on matters (such as privatization) that can be guaranteed to raise a head of political steam on both sides of the main political divide. In the process, public attention has been captivated much more by the ideological froth whipped up around the White Paper than by the deep and difficult issues of providing a balanced and efficient health service to an affluent, industrialized society in the late twentieth century. In the longer term, *Working for Patients* may be judged less by what it actually did than by what it forced out of the arena of public debate.

First, the White Paper placed on ice the issue of an appropriate level of funding for the NHS (even though it was exactly that debate which finally obliged the government to engage in its review of the service), and it effectively closed down the debate about the most appropriate ways of funding it. In this respect, the government was caught in 1991 in a web of its own spinning. Anxious not to be wounded politically by the opposition's accusations of its hidden intent to privatize the NHS, the Secretary of State persistently reiterated the government's unswerving commitment to a tax-funded service that remains (for the most part) free at the time of use. Yet however necessary this may have been politically, it suppressed a much needed debate on the wisdom of financing a modern health service in this way. Reliance upon central government funding and the minimization of user charges is not the only way of financing a modern health service and may not even be the best; but the alternatives came to be defined as prohibited areas of debate, even though many had expected them to form the centrepiece of the review group's deliberations. Consequently, and inevitably, the tensions between the expansive expectations of the public and the instinctive tendency of government towards fiscal restraint remained unresolved, surfacing in familiar ways in the first financial year following the White Paper's publication, and threatening to continue to do so into the future. All that may prove to have changed in this regard is the public perception of the source of blame: if hospital beds continue to close and creditors remain unpaid in order to avert an end-of-year deficit, it may become easier to deflect the finger of responsibility away from central government (and even from the RHAs and DHAs) towards the individual hospitals and other provider units who can stand accused of failing to deliver their contractual commitments within the prices they have negotiated.

Second, the White Paper avoided some uncomfortable issues of rationing by perpetuating the myth of a service that proceeds on the basis of planning for need. The core responsibility assigned to the commissioning agencies is that of assessing the needs of their resident populations and purchasing the services required to meet them. In reality, the NHS forwent the luxury of believing it was planning for need some 20 years ago, when the realization could be avoided no longer of the impossibility of satisfying everybody's needs for health care. The rhetoric notwithstanding, the real issue became that of spreading the fixed and finite resources available to the service in ways that were tolerably fair and productive of reasonably good results. The meeting of needs gave way to the rationing of resources, and to pretend otherwise was deception. The reversion to the language of needs assessment in *Working for Patients* not only fails to ring true (since the NHS will continue to be funded on an annual cash-limited basis that has nothing to do with meeting a specified amount of need but everything to do with the political and economic spirit of the times) but also shirks the tricky question of which services should be provided through the NHS and which should not. The pretence that a tax-funded health-care service can (and should) provide everything from cosmetic surgery to life-extending treatments must sooner or later be confronted for what it is. The NHS, financed as it is, cannot deliver all forms of health care of an acceptable standard to all who could benefit from them. Choices are inescapable, either about what is to be provided, or to whom, or at what standard. At present, such choices are exercised largely behind the veil of clinical autonomy, but the time may not be far off when an explicit distinction must be made between core services that will be delivered under guarantees of quality and timeliness to all who require them, and a secondary set that will not be available at all through the NHS or only to those who are willing to pay for them or who are defined in some other way.[3] If true, a public stage must be prepared upon which the arguments of ethics and morality can be rehearsed – no easy task, to be sure, but one that the White Paper fails even to recognize.

Third, the implementation of *Working for Patients* served to perpetuate the dilemma of whether the NHS is a central service that is locally managed or a local service operating within central guidelines. Governments have tended to claim the latter while actually willing the former. They cannot, for political reasons, remain indifferent to public perceptions of the performance of the NHS as a national service, but they have been increasingly willing to devolve responsibility for local shortcomings to the regions and districts. It seemed for a while that *Working for Patients* might constitute an important step towards the devolution of power: as depicted in the White Paper, the NHS trusts and the fund-holding general practices would hold important freedoms that could be exercised without the constricting interventions of central government. In the event, the prospect of such freedoms producing politically unacceptable outcomes proved too much for the government to bear, at least in the short term, and bureaucratic steps began to be taken to limit the very freedoms that had erstwhile been lauded as the keystones of the internal market. Meanwhile, the fragmentations and realignments within the districts were producing locally idiosyncratic service structures such that possibly no two districts were doing things in exactly the same way. The paradox was emerging of a health service looking increasingly less like a *national* health service while coming under the firm political control of central government. The perpetuation of the tensions between the centre and the periphery that have damaged the service in the past may continue to exercise their confounding influence into the brave new future.

There is no satisfactory point at which to draw the line across the balance sheet, for the momentous repercussions from *Working for Patients* will continue to echo for a long time to come. A true perspective will be open only to future historians of this extraordinary episode in the history of health care in the United Kingdom. The criteria they will use in reaching a balanced judgement may not even be known to contemporary commentators. Yet prophecy (in the biblical sense) has always been an honourable trade, and if helpful images of understanding can be seen in the mirror that this book has held up to our contemporary condition, then the labour will not have been in vain.

REFERENCES

Chapter 1 Origins

1 Bevan, A. (1952) *In Place of Fear*. London, Heinemann.
2 Perera, S. and Tirbutt, S. (1982) 'No trimming of policies prior to election' *The Guardian*, 9 October.
3 Green, D. G. (1986) *Challenge to the NHS*. London, Institute of Economic Affairs.
4 Peet, J. (1987) *Healthy Competition: How to Improve the NHS*. London, Centre for Policy Studies.
5 Conservative Central Office (1987) Full Speech by the Rt. Hon. John Moore MP . . . at the 104th Conservative Party Conference. London, Media Department, Conservative Central Office.
6 Cole, J. (1989) 'Capital care' *The Listener*, 9 February.
7 Judge, K., Smith, J. and Taylor-Gooby, P. (1983) 'Public opinion and the privatisation of welfare: some theoretical implications' *Journal of Social Policy*, 12, 469–89.
8 Robinson, R. and Judge, K. (1987) *Public Expenditure and the NHS: Trends and Prospects*. London, King's Fund Institute.
9 House of Commons Social Services Committee (1986) *Fourth Report 1985–6. Public Expenditure on the Social Services*, HC 387. London, HMSO.
10 House of Commons Social Services Committee (1988) *First Report 1987–8. Resourcing the National Health Service: Short Term Issues*, HC 264–1. London, HMSO.
11 House of Commons Treasury and Civil Service Committee (1988) *Second Report 1987–8. The Government's Expenditure Plans 1988–89 to 1990–91*, HC 292. London, HMSO.
12 Shocket, G. (1989) *Efficiency in the NHS: A Study of Cost Improvement Programmes*. London, King's Fund Institute, National Association of Health Authorities, and Institute of Health Service Management.
13 Mays, N. and Bevan, G. (1987) *Resource Allocation in the Health Service*. London, Bedford Square Press.

14 McKie, D. (1987) 'Mounting resistance to NHS cuts: disaster inevitable' *The Lancet*, 2, 752.
15 Timmins, N. (1988) *Cash, Crisis and Cure*. London, Newspaper Publishing plc.
16 Hoffenberg, R., Todd, I. P. and Pinker, G. (1987) 'Crisis in the National Health Service' *British Medical Journal*, 295, 1505.
17 Parliamentary Debates (1987) *House of Commons Official Report 1987–8*, vol. 24, col. 1094. London, HMSO.
18 Smith, T. (1988) 'New year message' *British Medical Journal*, 296, 1–2.
19 Parliamentary Debates (1988) *House of Commons Official Report 1987–8*, vol. 125, cols. 833–4. London, HMSO.
20 Webster, C. (1988) *The Health Services Since the War. Volume 1*. London, HMSO.
21 Farrell, C. (1980) 'The Royal Commission on the National Health Service' *Policy and Politics*, 8, 189–203.
22 Brown, C. (1989) 'Clarke braced for showdown over health review' *The Independent*, 30 January.
23 Davies, P. (1988) 'The public speaks out on the NHS' *Health Service Journal*, 98, 556–7.
24 Davies, P. (1988) 'How the NHS got £44 million without anyone noticing' *Health Service Journal*, 98, 264–5.
25 Timmins, N. (1990) '£55 million fund to speed NHS treatment fails' *The Independent*, 25 January.
26 Royal Commission on the National Health Service (1979) *Report*. Cmnd 7615. London, HMSO.
27 House of Commons Social Services Committee (1988) *Fifth Report 1987–8. The Future of the National Health Services*, HC 613. London, HMSO.
28 Ham, C., Robinson, R. and Benzeval, M. (1990) *Health Check*. London, King's Fund Institute.
29 Timmins, N. (1988) 'DHSS study urged end to tax-funded health care' *The Independent*, 8 February.
30 Brittan, L. (1988) *A New Deal for Health Care*. London, Conservative Political Centre.
31 Higgins, J. (1988) *The Business of Medicine*. London, Macmillan.
32 Leathley, A. (1989) 'Whatever happened to income generation?' *Health Service Journal*, 99, 1492–3.
33 Dean, M. (1990) 'An unhappy NHS fairy tale' *The Lancet*, 2, 1242–3.
34 Anon (1988) 'A national lottery to help fund the NHS' *The Lancet*, 1, 1007.
35 Pike, A. (1989) 'The health White Paper: review came amid row about shortages' *Financial Times*, 1 February.
36 Anon (1988) 'Half-bold on health: Britain's NHS will soon be reformed' *The Economist*, 17 December, 13.
37 Department of Health and Social Security (1983) *Health Care and its Costs*. London, HMSO.

38 National Audit Office (1986) *Value for Money Developments in the NHS*, HC 212. London, HMSO.
39 Jones, A. (1984) 'Seventy ways to cut costs' *Hospital and Health Services Review*, 80, 25–6.
40 House of Commons Committee of Public Accounts (1988) *Fifth Report 1987–8. Use of Operating Theatres in the National Health Service*, HC 348. London, HMSO.
41 Wilkin, D., Hallam, L., Leavey, R. and Metcalfe, D. (1987) *Anatomy of Urban General Practice*. London, Tavistock.
42 Public Finance Foundation (1988) *Financing the National Health Service*. London, Public Finance Foundation.
43 Green, D. G. (1988) *Everyone's a Private Patient*. London, Institute of Economic Affairs.
44 Anon (1988) 'A low cure for health' *The Economist*, 19 November, 37–8.
45 Brazier, J., Hutton, J. and Jeavons, R. (1990) *Analysing Health Care Systems: the Economic Context of the NHS White Paper Proposals*. York, Centre for Health Economics, University of York.

Chapter 2 Context

1 Department of Health and Social Security (1981) *Care in Action*. London, HMSO.
2 Parliamentary Debates (1991) *House of Commons Official Report 1990–1*, vol. 191, col. 413. London, HMSO.
3 Klein, R. (1989) *The Politics of the NHS*. London, Longman.
4 Hunter, D. J. (1991) 'Managing medicine: a response to the crisis' *Social Science and Medicine*, 32, 441–9.
5 Department of Health and Social Security (1972) *Management Arrangements for the Reorganised National Health Service*. London, HMSO.
6 Anon (1979) 'Tory health' *British Medical Journal*, 1, 1522.
7 Department of Health and Social Security (1979) *Patients First*. London, HMSO.
8 Parliamentary Debates (1983) *House of Commons Official Report 1983–4*, vol. 47, cols. 166–7. London, HMSO.
9 NHS Management Enquiry (1983) *Report*. London, Department of Health and Social Security.
10 Hardwick, R., de Bene, J. and Bussey, A. (1987) 'Doctors in management: three doctors' experiences' *British Medical Journal*, 194, 1498–9.
11 Department of Health and Social Security (1986) *Resource Management (Management Budgeting) in Health Authorities*, HN (86) 34. London, DHSS.
12 Packwood, T., Buxton, M. and Keen, J. (1990) 'Resource management in the National Health Service: a first case history' *Policy and Politics*, 18, 245–55.

13 Coombs, R., Bloomfield, B. and Rea, D. (1991) 'Differences in a scheme of change' *Health Service Journal*, 101, 16–17.
14 Masters, S. (1990) 'A natural evolution' *Health Service Journal*, 100, 555.
15 Anon (1989) 'Resource management' *Health Services Management*, 85, 53–4.
16 Perrin, J. (1988) *Resource Management in the NHS*. Wokingham, Van Nostrand Reinhold.
17 Buxton, M., Packwood, T. and Keen, J. (1991) *Final Report of the Brunel University Evaluation of Resource Management*. London, Health Economics Research Group, Brunel University.
18 Riddell, P. (1987) 'Plan to let NHS sell services' *Financial Times*, 25 November.
19 Department of Health (1989) *Income Generation: a Guide to Local Initiative*, HN (89)9. London, DH.
20 Moore, W. (1988) 'Beating private hospitals at their own game' *Health Service Journal*, 98, 904.
21 Pike, A. (1990) 'NHS – a new spirit lives' *Financial Times*, 29 January.
22 Leathley, A. (1989) 'Whatever happened to income generation?' *Health Service Journal*, 99, 1492.
23 Little, S. (1990) 'Experts fear bleak future for income generation' *Health Service Journal*, 100, 829.
24 Sheaff, R. (1991) *Marketing for Health Services*. Milton Keynes, Open University Press.
25 Timmins, N. (1987) 'Guy's agree deal for private firm to run pay-bed units' *The Independent*, 20 May.
26 Millar, B. (1987) 'Private profit comes to aid of public service' *Health Service Journal*, 97, 1372.
27 Timmins, N. (1988) 'NHS strikes more private health treatment deals' *The Independent*, 31 May.
28 Department of Health and Social Security (1983) *Competitive Tendering in the Provision of Domestic, Catering and Laundry Services*, HC (83) 18. London, DHSS.
29 Key, T. (1988) 'Contracting out ancillary services' in R. Maxwell (ed.) *Reshaping the National Health Service*. Hermitage, Policy Journals.
30 Timmins, N. (1987) 'Hospital building deal to save £3 million' *The Independent*, 3 November.
31 Tomkins, R. (1988) 'Midlands health service managers to buy out unit' *Financial Times*, 23 December.
32 Bunting, G. (1987) 'A not so sterile exercise' *Health Service Journal*, 97, 960–1.
33 Timmins, N. (1989) 'Pathology goes to tender' *The Independent*, 13 July.
34 Timmins, N. (1988) 'Fear of back-door privatisation of pathology service' *The Independent*, 12 January.

35 Dean, M. (1991) 'What happens after the election?' *The Lancet*, 337, 965–6.
36 Timmins, N. (1987) 'Hospitals want payment for treating outsiders' *The Independent*, 30 April.
37 Brazier, J. and Mays, N. (1987) 'Internal markets in NHS hospital care' *The Independent*, 5 May.
38 Timmins, N. (1988) 'NHS region may test internal market plan' *The Independent*, 14 March.
39 Moore, W. (1990) 'East Anglian RHA blazes the internal market trail' *Health Service Journal*, 100, 540.
40 Appleby, J., Middlemas, K. and Ranade, W. (1989) 'Provider markets: a glimpse of the future' *Health Service Journal*, 99, 414–15.
41 Ware, J. E. *et al.* (1986) 'Comparison of health outcomes at a health maintenance organisation with those of fee-for-service care' *The Lancet*, 1, 1017–22.
42 Saltman, R. B. (1990) 'Competition and reform in the Swedish health system' *Milbank Memorial Fund Quarterly*, 68, 597–618.
43 Dekker, W. (1987) *Bereidheid tot Verandering*. Amsterdam, Commissie Structuur en Financiering Gezondheidszorg.
44 Davies, P. (1989) 'Setting an example in New Zealand' *Health Service Journal*, 99, 68–9.
45 Anon (1989) 'Cuts in New Zealand' *British Medical Journal*, 298, 1668–9.
46 Deardon, B. (1991) 'First welfare state at the end of the road' *Health Service Journal*, 8 August, 15.
47 Marinker, M. (1984) 'Developments in primary health care' in G. Teeling Smith (ed.) *A New NHS Act for 1996?* London, Office of Health Economics.
48 Enthoven, A. C. (1985) *Reflections on the Management of the National Health Service*. London, Nuffield Provincial Hospitals Trust.
49 Roberts, J. (1990) 'Kenneth Clarke: hatchet man or remoulder?' *British Medical Journal*, 301, 1383–6.
50 Department of Health and Social Security (1986) *Review of the RAWP Formula*. London, DHSS.
51 Timmins, N. (1988) 'PM to encourage changes in NHS internal market' *The Independent*, 26 January.
52 Robinson, R. (1988) *Efficiency and the NHS: A Case for Internal Markets*. London, Institute of Economic Affairs Health Unit.
53 Anon (1988) 'Competing prescriptions: proposals for structural changes in the NHS' *The Economist*, 27 February, 306.
54 House of Commons Social Services Committee (1988) *Fifth Report 1987–8. The Future of the National Health Service*, HC 613. London, HMSO.
55 Laurance, J. (1989) 'Health service faces top-to-toe overhaul' *The Sunday Times*, 22 January.

Chapter 3 Content

1 Secretaries of State for Health, Wales, Northern Ireland and Scotland (1989) *Working for Patients*, Cmnd 555. London, HMSO.
2 Department of Health (1989) *NHS Review Working Papers*. (1) Self-governing hospitals. (2) Funding and contracts for health services. (3) Practice budgets for general medical practitioners. (4) Indicative prescribing budgets for general medical practitioners. (5) Capital charges. (6) Medical audit. (7) NHS consultants: appointments, contracts and distinction awards. (8) Implications for family practitioner committees. London, HMSO.
3 Richards, S. (1989) 'The course of cultural change' *Health Service Journal*, 99, Supplement, 1–2.
4 Millar, B. (1989) 'Healthwatch UK: the TV spectacular' *Health Service Journal*, 99, 169.
5 Davies, P. (1989) 'The show must go on, whatever the cost' *Health Service Journal*, 99, 1241.
6 Sherman, J. (1989) 'Clarke says BMA leaflet misleading' *The Times*, 20 April.
7 Dean, M. (1990) 'Uncertain future of the NHS' *The Lancet*, 336, 105–6.
8 Department of Health and Social Security (1983) *Competitive Tendering in the Provision of Domestic, Catering and Laundry Services*, HC (83) 18. London, DHSS.
9 Enthoven, A. C. (1985) *Reflections on the Management of the National Health Service*. London, Nuffield Provincial Hospitals Trust.
10 Roberts, J. (1990) 'Kenneth Clarke: hatchet man or remoulder?' *British Medical Journal*, 301, 1383–6.
11 Marinker, M. (1984) 'Developments in primary health care' in G. Teeling Smith (ed.) *A New NHS Act for 1996?* London, Office of Health Economics.
12 Anon (1988) 'A slow cure for health' *The Economist*, 19 November, 37–8.
13 Brown, C. (1988) 'Family doctors get key role in reformed NHS' *The Independent*, 28 December.
14 Lewis, J. (1989) 'Mr Clarke defends his review' *The Lancet*, 1, 453.
15 House of Commons Social Services Committee (1988) *Fifth Report 1987–8. The Future of the National Health Service*, HC 613. London, HMSO.
16 Timmins, N. (1988) 'Government aims to let NHS hospitals opt out' *The Independent*, 5 December.
17 Pike, A. (1989) 'Hospitals weigh prognosis for opting out' *Financial Times*, 24 January.
18 Millar, B. (1989) 'What about a little self control?' *Health Service Journal*, 99, 70.
19 Hunter, D. J. (1989) 'First define your terms' *Health Service Journal*, 99, 1475.

20 Ham, C. and Best, G. (1989) 'Goodbye rubber stamp image' *Health Service Journal*, 99, 482–3.
21 Tomlin, Z. (1991) 'Whistling down the wind' *Health Service Journal*, 12 December, 14.
22 Department of Health and Social Security (1976) *Sharing Resources for Health in England*. London, HMSO.
23 Department of Health and Social Security (1988) *Review of Resource Allocation Working Party Formula: Final Report of the NHS Management Board*. London, DHSS.
24 Robinson, R. (1989) 'New health care market' *British Medical Journal*, 298, 437–9.
25 MacPherson, G. (1989) 'No cash limits for GPs' drug budgets' *British Medical Journal*, 299, 875–6.
26 Anon (1989) 'Mr Clarke's prescription' *Financial Times*, 1 February.
27 Anon (1989) 'Hospitals set free' *The Economist*, 4 February, 17–18.
28 Laing, W. (1989) 'The White Paper and the independent sector: scope for growth and restructuring' *British Medical Journal*, 298, 821–3.
29 Timmins, N. (1989) 'Hospitals will be encouraged to opt out' *The Independent*, 5 January.
30 Stephens, P. (1989) 'MPs return to a health debate: the politics of the NHS' *Financial Times*, 10 January.
31 Davies, P. (1989) 'MPs weigh in for health bill debate' *Health Service Journal*, 99, 194.
32 NHS Management Executive (1989) *Contracts for Health Services: Operational Principles*, EL (89) MB 1169. London, Department of Health.
33 Davies, P. (1989) 'White Paper show – with no support act' *Health Service Journal*, 99, 223.
34 Anon (1990) 'Treatment suspended' *The Economist*, 16 June, 33.

Chapter 4 Purposes

1 Lock, S. (1989) 'Pride and prejudice' *British Medical Journal*, 298, 1197.
2 Parliamentary Debates (1988) *House of Commons Official Report 1987–8*, vol. 125, cols 833–4. London, HMSO.
3 Aitken, I. (1989) 'Hoist signals and stand by to go about' *The Guardian*, 26 June.
4 Brindle, D. and Linton, M. (1989) 'Survey shows health service plans will lose Tory votes' *The Guardian*, 10 October.
5 Secretary of State for Social Services (1972) *National Health Service Reorganisation: England*, Cmnd. 5055. London, HMSO.
6 Smith, T. (1989) 'BMA rejects NHS review but doctors must develop a coherent alternative' *British Medical Journal*, 298, 1405–6.
7 Anon (1988) 'Half-hold on health' *The Economist*, 17 December, 13.

8 Laurance, J. and Hughes, D. (1989) 'Clarke promises to stay flat out on NHS reforms' *The Sunday Times*, 7 May.
9 Anon (1989) 'All to play for, says minister' *Health Service Journal*, 99, 159.
10 Mason, J. (1989) 'Return to two-tier care feared – NHS reform' *Financial Times*, 19 April.
11 Nettleton, P. (1989) 'Owen says Tories are creating 1930s-style health system' *The Guardian*, 19 April.
12 Pike, A. (1989) 'Kenneth Clarke, Health Secretary, replies to critics of his proposals to reform the NHS' *Financial Times*, 11 April.
13 Warden, J. (1989) 'Clarke steps out' *British Medical Journal*, 298, 1478.
14 Mellor, D. (1989) 'Why there is no choice but change' *Financial Times*, 30 August.
15 Roberts, J. (1990) 'Kenneth Clarke: hatchet man or remoulder?' *British Medical Journal*, 301, 1383–6.
16 Glasman, D. (1991) 'Prepare to run before stormy winds of change' *Health Service Journal*, 24 January, 12.
17 Smith, R. (1991) 'William Waldegrave: thinking on the new NHS' *British Medical Journal*, 302, 636–40.
18 Ham, C. and Best, G. (1989) 'Goodbye rubber stamp image' *Health Service Journal*, 99, 482–3.
19 Davidson, N. (1989) 'After the battles, time to talk business' *Health Service Journal*, 99, 879.
20 NHS Management Executive (1990) 'Trusts must get financial management right' *NHSME News*, 38, 8.
21 Lewis, J. (1989) 'Mr Clarke defends his review' *The Lancet*, 1, 453.
22 Bottomley, V. (1991) Speech to Conference of Institute of Health Service Management and National Association of Health Authorities and Trusts, 4 March. London, Department of Health.
23 Willetts, D. (1989) 'The NHS remedy – to be taken internally' *The Guardian*, 1 February.
24 Lock, S. (1989) 'Steaming through the NHS' *British Medical Journal*, 298, 619–20.
25 Anon (1989) 'Dr Whinge, QC' *The Economist*, 18 March, 51–2.
26 Phillips, M. (1989) 'Cheap cracks and common concern' *The Guardian*, 10 March.
27 Timmins, N. (1989) 'Is the NHS safe in their hands?' *The Independent*, 9 February.
28 MacPherson, G. (1989) 'BMA's measured response' *British Medical Journal*, 298, 340–1.
29 Anon (1989) 'Slow down, Mr Clarke' *Financial Times*, 11 August.
30 Stephens, P. (1989) 'Clarke to seek further NHS funds' *Financial Times*, 1 February.
31 Warden, J. (1990) 'Beginning of the end of state NHS' *British Medical Journal*, 301, 199.

32 Pike, A. (1989) 'The health White Paper: reading between the lines to find future of NHS' *Financial Times*, 1 February.
33 Maynard, A. (1989) *Whither the National Health Service?* York, Centre for Health Economics, University of York.
34 Prowse, M. (1989) 'Competitors in white coats: the economics underlying public concern at the government's plans for the NHS' *Financial Times*, 22 August.
35 Currie, C. (1989) 'Dr Owen on the White Paper' *British Medical Journal*, 299, 1243–4.
36 Jenkins, P. (1989) 'Doctors draw the political battle lines' *The Independent*, 21 March.
37 Brown, C. (1989) 'Clarke refuses to back down to GPs' *The Independent*, 14 March.
38 Anon (1989) 'Clarke urges Tory MPs to counter misinformation' *The Independent*, 15 March.

Chapter 5 Dissent

1 Timmins, N. (1989) 'Doctors set to campaign against changes in NHS' *The Independent*, 28 January.
2 Beecham, L. (1989) 'GMSC to consider concept of GP budgets' *British Medical Journal*, 298, 259.
3 Anon (1989) 'BMA misgivings at price on patients' *The Times*, 1 February.
4 Hall, C. (1989) 'A boyish Dr Clarke sugars the pill' *The Independent*, 2 February.
5 Timmins, N. (1989) 'Doctors to mount campaign against NHS reform plans' *The Independent*, 3 March.
6 Dewhurst, J. K. (1989) 'NHS review' *British Medical Journal*, 298, 400.
7 Anon (1989) 'Calls for GPs to resign from NHS' *British Medical Journal*, 298, 759–60.
8 Brindle, D. (1989) 'GPs revolt on plans for reform' *The Guardian*, 9 March.
9 Timmins, N. and Hall, C. (1989) 'GPs threaten to quit over health review' *The Independent*, 9 March.
10 Brindle, D. (1989) 'Forget your wallets, Clarke tells doctors' *The Guardian*, 10 March.
11 Hall, C. (1989) 'Family doctors launch SOS for the NHS fight' *The Independent*, 1 April.
12 Timmins, N. (1989) 'Nurses' college joins NHS reform protest' *The Independent*, 17 March.
13 Sherman, J. (1989) 'Clarke is accused of undermining NHS principles' *The Times*, 5 April.
14 Beecham, L. (1989) 'Juniors warn White Paper will not help patients' *British Medical Journal*, 298, 756–9.

15 Anon (1989) 'Resource management pilot schemes' *British Medical Journal*, 298, 979.
16 Ballantyne, A. (1989) 'Consultants spurn hospital opt-outs' *The Guardian*, 21 March.
17 Sherman, J. (1989) 'Ignore pressure to opt out, BMA says' *The Times*, 10 April.
18 Anon (1989) 'CCHMS launches initiative on self governing hospitals' *British Medical Journal*, 298, 1256–7.
19 Warden, J. (1989) 'GPs make MPs bristle' *British Medical Journal*, 298, 1059.
20 Parliamentary Debates (1989) *House of Commons Official Report 1987–8*, vol. 151, col. 788. London, HMSO.
21 Anon (1989) 'GPs attack White Paper' *British Medical Journal*, 298, 1316–19.
22 Timmins, N. (1989) 'GPs resist resignation over NHS proposals' *The Independent*, 28 April.
23 Anon (1989) 'From the Special Representative Meeting' *British Medical Journal*, 298, 1455–7.
24 Lowry, S. (1989) 'BMA – working for patients, with a mandate' *British Medical Journal*, 298, 1411–12.
25 Sherman, J. (1989) 'Clarke attacks BMA scare adverts on reforms' *The Times*, 19 May.
26 Timmins, N. (1989) 'Doctors' new posters take NHS protest bill to £1.9 million' *The Independent*, 27 July.
27 Anon (1989) 'Dangerous doctors' *The Economist*, 19 August, 19–20.
28 Brown, C. (1989) 'Minister stakes his future on a high-risk strategy' *The Independent*, 5 July.
29 National Audit Office (1989) *Financial Management in the National Health Service*, HC 566. London, HMSO.
30 House of Commons Social Services Committee (1989) *Fifth Report 1988–9. Resourcing the National Health Service: The Government's White Paper; Working For Patients*, HC 214–II. London, HMSO.
31 Anon (1990) 'GMSC chairman warns GPs on budget holding' *British Medical Journal*, 300, 1469–70.
32 Dyer, C. (1989) 'Have a go consultants get high court go ahead' *British Medical Journal*, 299, 1482.
33 Prentice, T. (1989) 'Doctor puts house on line in fight against NHS reforms' *The Times*, 30 December.
34 Delamothe, T. (1989) 'New party to contest marginal seats over government's plans for the NHS' *British Medical Journal*, 299, 1481.
35 Kellner, P. (1991) 'Patients place their faith in the NHS' *The Independent*, 22 July.
36 Beecham, L. (1990) 'BMA continues to oppose damaging effects of NHS bill' *British Medical Journal*, 300, 126–8.
37 Beecham, L. (1990) 'MPs to be told of JCC's worries on NHS bill' *British Medical Journal*, 330, 334–5.

38 Anon (1990) 'GPs overwhelmingly oppose trusts' *British Medical Journal*, 301, 782.
39 O'Sullivan, J. (1990) 'Clarke responds to BMA by urging all hospitals to opt out' *The Independent*, 19 September.
40 Brahams, D. (1990) 'NHS reforms: doctor's legal challenge fails' *The Lancet*, 335, 528–9.
41 Anon (1990) 'NHS reforms: BMA should raise profile' *British Medical Journal*, 301, 933–5.
42 Smith, J. R. (1991) 'The BMA in agony' *British Medical Journal*, 303, 74.
43 Anon (1991) 'BMA council chairman criticised' *British Medical Journal*, 303, 76–7.
44 Anon (1991) 'NHS reforms' *British Medical Journal*, 303, 128.
45 Klein, R. (1991) 'The politics of change' *British Medical Journal*, 302, 1102–3.
46 Anon (1989) 'Medicine and the market' *Financial Times*, 21 April.
47 Beecham, L. (1989) 'Triumph of hope over experience' *British Medical Journal*, 298, 1103–4.
48 Laurent, C. (1989) 'Church versus state: the White Paper clash' *Health Service Journal*, 99, 1026.
49 National Consumer Council (1989) *NCC Response to the Secretary of State for Health*. London, National Consumer Council.
50 Office of Health Economics (1989) *Measurement and Management in the NHS*. London, Office of Health Economics.
51 Green, D. G. (ed.) (1990) *The NHS Reforms: Whatever Happened to Consumer Choice?* London, IEA Health and Welfare Unit.
52 Timmins, N. (1989) 'Clarke admits that doctors are winning battle on NHS plans' *The Independent*, 5 July.
53 Anon (1990) 'Poll confirms public still opposes NHS review' *British Medical Journal*, 300, 685.
54 Boseley, S. (1990) 'The new commercial battleground for patient care' *The Guardian*, 27 June.
55 Timmins, N. (1989) 'Guy's pushes for self-government' *The Independent*, 2 February.
56 Moore, W. (1991) 'Survey shows managers cool over NHS reforms' *Health Service Journal*, 13 June, 101.
57 Anon (1989) 'Budget proposals divide family doctors' *The Independent*, 4 February.
58 Lilford, R. (1989) 'Looking to a better future' *Health Service Journal*, 99, 1190–1.
59 Chantler, C. (1990) 'Medicine and politics' *British Medical Journal*, 300, 124.
60 Sheldon, T. (1989) 'Doctors set up group to back White Paper' *Health Service Journal*, 99, 1449.
61 Jenkins, S. (1989) 'A savage attack of hypochondria' *The Sunday Times*, 16 April.

62 Mellor, D. (1989) 'Why there is no choice but change' *Financial Times*, 30 August.
63 Beecham, L. (1989) 'BMA launches campaign against White Paper' *British Medical Journal*, 298, 676–7.
64 Royal College of Physicians (1989) *Medical Audit: What, Why and How?* London, Royal College of Physicians of London.
65 Conference of Medical Royal Colleges and Their Faculties in the UK (1989) *Building on the White Paper. Some Suggestions and Safeguards*. London, Royal College of Physicians of London.
66 Anon (1989) 'Public opposition to White Paper increases' *British Medical Journal*, 299, 863.
67 House of Commons Social Services Committee (1990) *First Report 1989–90*, HC 665. London, HMSO.
68 National Association of Health Authorities and Trusts (1991) *Spring Financial Survey 1991*. Birmingham, NAHAT.
69 Robinson, R. and Judge, K. (1987) *Public Expenditure and the NHS: Trends and Prospects*. London, King's Fund Institute.
70 Chartered Institute of Public Finance and Accountancy (1989) *Health Service Trends 1989. Volume 1*. London, CIPFA.
71 Griffiths, R. (1988) *Community Care. Agenda for Action*. London, HMSO.
72 Anon (1989) 'Hospitals set free' *The Economist*, 4 February, 17–18.
73 Kafetz, K. (1989) 'Tell me the old, old story' *The Guardian*, 13 February.
74 Anon (1989) 'Standing Committee on Postgraduate Medical Education disquieted by threats to training' *British Medical Journal*, 299, 509.

Chapter 6 Prophecies

1 Anon (1989) 'All to play for, says minister' *Health Service Journal*, 99, 159.
2 Robinson, R. (1990) *Competition and Health Care. A Comparative Analysis of UK Plans and US Experience*. London, King's Fund Institute.
3 Shroeder, S. A. and Cantor, J. C. (1991) 'Cost control fails again' *New England Journal of Medicine*, 325, 1099–1100.
4 Dean, M. (1990) 'Will the doctors opt out?' *The Lancet*, 335, 341–2.
5 Herzlinger, R. E. (1989) 'The failed revolution in health care – the role of management' *Harvard Business Review*, March–April, 95–103.
6 Prowse, M. (1990) 'Rewriting the NHS rule book' *Financial Times*, 19 January.
7 Glasman, D. (1990) 'Managers start exodus from purchasing role' *Health Service Journal*, 101, 1409.
8 Department of Health (1990) *Developing Districts*. London, HMSO.
9 Crump, B., Drummond, M. and Marchment, M. (1990) 'The DGM's dilemma' *Health Service Journal*, 100, 552–3.

10 Moore, W. (1990) 'Purchaser–provider split makes trusts inevitable' *Health Service Journal*, 100, 271.
11 Ham, C. (1990) *Holding On While Letting Go*. London, King's Fund Institute.
12 Department of Health (1989) *Pricing the Openness in Contracts for Health Services*. London, DH.
13 Roberts, H. and Robinson, R. (1989) 'Health at what price?' *Health Service Journal*, 99, 1511.
14 Appleby, J., Middlemas, K. and Ranade, W. (1989) 'Provider markets: a glimpse of the future' *Health Service Journal*, 99, 414–15.
15 Timmins, N. (1989) 'Doctors sceptical after trial pricing of NHS treatment' *The Independent*, 14 March.
16 Mellor, D. (1989) 'Why there is no choice but change' *Financial Times*, 30 August.
17 Anon (1989) 'Calculated Chaos' *The Guardian*, 30 November.
18 Maynard, A. (1990) 'First consult your lawyer' *Health Service Journal*, 100, 404.
19 Stocking, B. (1989) 'Setting the standard' *Health Service Journal*, 99, 1470–1.
20 Hopkins, A. and Maxwell, R. (1990) 'Contracts and quality of care' *British Medical Journal*, 300, 919–22.
21 National Health Service Management Executive (1990) *Contracts for Health Services: Operating Contracts*. London, HMSO.
22 Powell, M. (1991) 'Contracts of a clinical kind' *Health Service Journal*, 1 August, 18–19.
23 Anon (1989) 'Slow down, Mr Clarke' *Financial Times*, 11 August.
24 Glasman, D. (1990) 'Disillusioned health chiefs quit over reforms' *Health Service Journal*, 100, 751.
25 Ham, C. and Hunter, D. (1988) *Managing Clinical Activity in the NHS*. London, King's Fund Institute.
26 Beecham, L. (1989) 'LMCs call to stop White Paper talks rejected' *British Medical Journal*, 298, 53–5.
27 Smith, R. (1989) 'Words from the source: an interview with Alain Enthoven' *British Medical Journal*, 298, 1166–8.
28 Smedley, E. *et al.* (1989) *A Costing Analysis of General Practice Budgets*. York, Centre for Health Economics, University of York.
29 Anon (1989) 'Mr Clarke's colander' *The Guardian*, 14 December.
30 May, A. (1989) 'A guru vexed by his government disciples' *Health Service Journal*, 99, 1150.
31 Scheffler, R. (1989) 'Adverse selection: the Achilles heel of the NHS reforms' *The Lancet*, 1, 950–2.
32 Maynard, A. (1989) *Whither the National Health Service?* York, Centre for Health Economics, University of York.
33 Atkinson, C. (1989) 'Donning a manager's cap' *Health Service Journal*, 99, 1218–19.

34 Cocks, I. (1990) 'General practice budget holding' *British Medical Journal*, 300, 1017–18.
35 Beecham, L. (1990) 'MPs to be told of JCC's worries on NHS bill' *British Medical Journal*, 300, 334–5.
36 Ford, J. C. (1990) 'General practice fundholders' *British Medical Journal*, 300, 1027–8.
37 Enthoven, A. C. (1985) *Reflections on the Management of the National Health Service*. London, Nuffield Provincial Hospitals Trust.
38 National Health Service Management Executive (1989) *Contracts for Health Services: Operational Principles*, EL (89) MB 169. London, Department of Health.
39 Millar, B. (1990) 'Emerging from the golden chrysalis' *Health Service Journal*, 100, 1720–1.
40 Cook, H. (1989) 'The price of freedom' *Health Service Journal*, 99, 364–5.
41 Millar, B. (1990) 'Consciousness raising on capital costs' *Health Service Journal*, 99, 381.
42 Sheldon, T. (1989) 'Inner London worst hit under internal market' *Health Service Journal*, 99, 1020.
43 Bryan, S. (1989) 'Charging into confusion' *Health Service Journal*, 99, 818–19.
44 Green, D. (1989) 'A step in the right direction' *Health Service Journal*, 99, 168.
45 Moore, W. (1989) 'Patients' groups demand White Paper pilot studies' *Health Service Journal*, 99, 627.
46 Beecham, L. (1989) 'BMA launches campaign against White Paper' *British Medical Journal*, 298, 676–9.
47 Davies, P. (1989) 'Where will the money come from and go to?' *Health Service Journal*, 99, 477.
48 Tomlin, Z. (1989) 'Pay beds add to waiting lists, claims Yates' *Health Service Journal*, 101, 3.
49 Davies, P. (1991) 'An unwanted critic on the waiting list' *Health Service Journal*, 14 March, 15.
50 Millar, B. (1990) 'Up in the air after a smooth takeoff' *Health Service Journal*, 100, 1105.
51 Anon (1990) 'Contracts' *Health Services Management*, 86, 5.
52 Timmins, N. (1989) 'Deals for operations bring good news and a bad joke' *The Independent*, 28 December.
53 Brindle, D. (1989) 'The year ahead – health' *The Guardian*, 5 January.
54 Warden, J. (1990) 'Chairman Clarke's message' *British Medical Journal*, 300, 217.
55 Delamothe, T. (1990) 'GP fundholding' *British Medical Journal*, 301, 1009.
56 Anon (1990) 'IHA calls for split contracts' *Health Service Journal*, 100, 1273.
57 Jones, T. (1989) 'What they left out' *Health Service Journal*, 99, 1368–9.

58 Laing, W. (1989) 'The White Paper and the independent sector: scope for growth and restructuring' *British Medical Journal*, 298, 821–3.
59 Lee, P. R. and Etheredge, L. (1989) 'Clinical freedom: two lessons for the UK from the US experience with privatisation of health care' *The Lancet*, 1, 263–5.
60 National Health Service Management Executive (1989) 'Framework for information and IT Working paper'. Draft of 4.12.89. London, Department of Health.
61 Warden, J. (1989) 'No clues from Clarke on NHS review' *British Medical Journal*, 298, 777–8.
62 Appleby, J. (1990) 'Information overload?' *British Medical Journal*, 300, 419.
63 Barr, N., Glennerster, H. and Le Grand, J. (1989) 'Working for Patients: The right approach' *Social Policy and Administration*, 23, 117–27.
64 Pike, A. (1989) 'Survey of health care: responding in metaphors' *Financial Times*, 11 April.
65 Anon (1989) 'GPs attack White Paper' *British Medical Journal*, 298, 1316–19.
66 Prowse, M. (1989) 'Why Britain's doctors are up in arms' *Financial Times*, 22 March.
67 Lewis, J. (1989) 'Mr Clarke defends his review' *The Lancet*, 1, 453.
68 Brindle, D. (1989) 'Opting-out hospitals may be free to drop some services' *The Guardian*, 22 April.
69 Anon (1989) 'Opposition peers fiercely critical' *The Times*, 1 February.
70 Smith, R. (1991) 'William Waldegrave: thinking on the new NHS' *British Medical Journal*, 302, 636–40.
71 Sheldon, T. (1990) 'No accounting for secrecy over costs' *Health Service Journal*, 100, 1064.
72 Pollitt, C. (1989) 'Consuming passions' *Health Service Journal*, 99, 1436–7.
73 Brindle, D. (1990) 'Secret plan to ease in hospital opt-outs' *The Guardian*, 17 April.
74 Maclachlan, R. (1990) 'CHCs defeated in fight to win more power' *Health Service Journal*, 100, 1053.
75 Maclachlan, R. (1990) 'Continuing to advocate against all the odds' *Health Service Journal*, 100, 1062.
76 Delamothe, T. (1990) 'Hey, big spender' *British Medical Journal*, 300, 286.
77 Sims, J. (1989) 'GPs force college to reject damaging White Paper' *Health Service Journal*, 99, 468.
78 Anon (1989) 'From the Special Representative Meeting' *British Medical Journal*, 298, 1455–7.
79 Brown, C. (1989) 'Clarke urged to investigate GPs' services' *The Independent*, 29 December.

Chapter 7 Implementation

1 Anon (1990) 'Treatment suspended' *The Economist*, 16 June, 33.
2 Ellis, N. (1989) 'Outline of proposed package of changes to GPs' contracts' *British Medical Journal*, 298, 1387–9.
3 Timmins, N. (1989) 'GPs to fight imposition of contract' *The Independent*, 7 March.
4 Timmins, N. (1989) 'More doctors in threat to quit over reforms' *The Independent*, 11 March.
5 Laurance, J. and Hughes, D. (1989) 'Clarke promises to stay flat out on NHS reforms' *The Sunday Times*, 7 May.
6 Anon (1989) 'Contract changes to be commended to GPs' *British Medical Journal*, 298, 1271.
7 Anon (1989) 'Minister imposes GPs' contract as GMSC holds special meeting' *British Medical Journal*, 299, 461–2.
8 Warden, J. (1989) 'Clarke steps out' *British Medical Journal*, 298, 1478.
9 Timmins, N. (1988) 'NHS urged to draw up patient care contracts' *The Independent*, 19 April.
10 Bevan, G., Holland, W., Maynard, A. and Mays, N. (1988) *Reforming UK Health Care to Improve Health*. York, Centre for Health Economics, University of York.
11 Timmins, N. (1988) 'NHS region may test internal market plan' *The Independent*, 14 March.
12 Anon (1989) 'BMA checklist for government's NHS review' *British Medical Journal*, 298, 124.
13 Smith, R. (1989) 'Words from the source: an interview with Alain Enthoven' *British Medical Journal*, 298, 1166–8.
14 Timmins, N. (1989) 'Clarke softens NHS tone' *The Independent*, 25 May.
15 Davies, P. (1989) 'Ready for take-off without the pilots' *Health Service Journal*, 99, 662.
16 Beecham, L. (1989) 'BMA launches campaign against White Paper' *British Medical Journal*, 298, 676–9.
17 Brindle, D. (1989) 'Pace being forced in health service shake-up' *The Guardian*, 13 March.
18 Millar, B. (1989) 'FPCs voice fears over White Paper timetable' *Health Service Journal*, 99, 374.
19 Appleby, J. (1989) 'Accountants question Working for Patients' *British Medical Journal*, 298, 1271–2.
20 House of Commons Social Services Committee (1989) *Fifth Report 1988–9. Resourcing the National Health Service: The Government's White Paper; Working for Patients*, HC 214–II. London, HMSO.
21 Lock, S. (1989) 'Steaming through the NHS' *British Medical Journal*, 298. 619–20.
22 Brindle, D. (1989) 'Clarke stresses opt-out hospitals must win staff and local support' *The Guardian*, 6 February.

23 Anon (1989) 'Limited support among doctors for self governing hospitals' *British Medical Journal*, 298, 1650–2.
24 House of Commons Social Services Committee (1989) *Fifth Report 1988–9. Resourcing the National Health Service: The Government's White Paper; Working for Patients*, HC 214. London, HMSO.
25 Timmins, N. (1989) 'Clarke gives extra cash for teaching and research' *The Independent*, 11 July.
26 Beecham, L. (1990) 'Survey shows consultants oppose NHS trusts' *British Medical Journal*, 300, 403–4.
27 Beecham, L. (1990) 'Mutiny on the flagship, but only a third vote' *British Medical Journal*, 300, 417–18.
28 De Bruxelles, S. (1990) 'Bart's upsets opt-out plan for hospitals' *The Observer*, 8 April.
29 Delamothe, T. (1990) 'Consultants say no to self-governing trusts' *British Medical Journal*, 300, 1539.
30 Warden, J. (1990) 'Trusting in Mr Clarke' *British Medical Journal*, 301, 81.
31 Dean, M. (1990) 'Manicures and Chablis but no extra NHS cash' *The Lancet*, 336, 995–6.
32 Warden, J. (1989) 'The White Paper has lift off' *British Medical Journal*, 298, 409–10.
33 Anon (1989) 'On course with the strategy, reports GMSC chairman' *British Medical Journal*, 298, 1185–7.
34 Millar, B. (1989) 'White Paper innovators – jumping the gun?' *Health Service Journal*, 99, 566.
35 Anon (1989) 'Minister offers scant reassurance to medical managers' *British Medical Journal*, 298, 1321–2.
36 Tillett, R. (1989) 'White Paper fears' *The Independent*, 24 May.
37 Timmins, N. (1989) 'Consultants threatened over hospital opt-out votes' *The Independent*, 17 June.
38 Bradford, W. P. (1989) 'Mr Clarke's willing volunteers' *British Medical Journal*, 298, 1641–2.
39 Weatherall, D. (1989) 'Hospitals, research and medical teaching' *The Independent*, 17 May.
40 Glasman, D. (1991) 'First the dream – now comes the reality' *Health Service Journal*, 14 February, 14.
41 Anon (1989) 'Mr Clarke's colander' *The Guardian*, 14 December.
42 Department of Health (1989) *Funding General Practice*. London, DH.
43 White, C. (1990) 'Computers and GP fundholders' *British Medical Journal*, 301, 893.
44 Department of Health (1990) *Developing Districts*. London, HMSO.
45 Hunt, L. (1990) 'Tory appointments turning NHS into a one-party state' *The Independent*, 15 October.
46 Anon (1989) 'Unforeseen mergers' *Health Service Journal*, 99, 1389.
47 Anon (1990) 'The future role of health authorities' *Health Services Management*, 86, 50.

48 Liddell, A. and Parston, G. (1990) 'How the market crashed' *Health Service Journal*, 100, 730–2.
49 Moore, W. (1989) 'FPC and community may merge if Guy's opt out' *Health Service Journal*, 99, 933.
50 Sheldon, T. (1990) 'More HAs link up in joint purchasing moves' *Health Service Journal*, 100, 1799.
51 National Health Service Management Executive (1991) *Integrating Primary and Secondary Health Care*. London, Department of Health.
52 Maynard, A. (1990) 'Danger ahead?' *Health Service Journal*, 100, 1611.
53 Lynch, T. (1989) 'Cook attacks choice of industrialists for NHS Policy Board' *Financial Times*, 24 May.
54 Warden, J. (1990) 'Shaping tomorrow's world' *British Medical Journal*, 300, 897.
55 Moore, W. (1991) 'Clean sweep needed to put house in order' *Health Service Journal*, 7 March, 14.
56 Klein, R. (1990) 'What future for the Department of Health?' *British Medical Journal*, 301, 481–4.
57 Sheldon, T. (1990) 'When it makes sense to mince your words' *Health Service Journal*, 100, 1211.
58 Brindle, D. (1990) 'Waldegrave shuns business jargon' *The Guardian*, 13 December.
59 Beecham, L. (1991) 'Taking the bureaucracy out of the GP contract' *British Medical Journal*, 302, 367.
60 Anon (1991) 'Health and education reforms – half right' *The Economist*, 9 February, 43–4.
61 O'Sullivan, J. (1991) 'NHS secret offer by doctors' *The Independent*, 1 June.
62 O'Sullivan, J. (1990) 'Hospitals planning to opt out could go bankrupt' *The Independent*, 9 October.
63 Glasman, D. (1991) 'First the dream – now comes the reality' *Health Service Journal*, 14 February, 14.
64 Ferriman, A. (1991) 'Doctors accuse government of lying' *The Observer*, 24 March.
65 O'Sullivan, J. (1991) 'District short of cash for patient referrals' *The Independent*, 20 June.
66 Scheuer, M. A. and Robinson, R. (1991) 'A wild card in the pack?' *Health Service Journal*, 8 August, 18–20.
67 Jones, J. (1991) 'GPs agree to truce in dispute over NHS' *The Independent*, 20 June.
68 Brindle, D. (1990) 'Bed closures force health cash U-turn' *The Guardian*, 19 December.
69 Hunt, L. and Jones, J. (1991) 'Two trust hospitals plan to cut 900 jobs' *The Independent*, 27 April.
70 Moore, W. (1991) 'Guy's and doles and local polls' *Health Service Journal*, 16 May, 13.

71 O'Sullivan, J. (1991) 'Health commission must face century-old problems' *The Independent*, 10 October.

Chapter 8 Reflections

1 Anon (1990) 'A duty to the facts' *Health Service Journal*, 100, 689.
2 Department of Health and Social Security (1979) *Patients First*. London, HMSO.
3 British Medical Association (1991) *Leading for Health. A BMA Agenda for Health*. London, BMA.

INDEX